Translational Medicine Research

Series editors

Translational medicine converts promising laboratory discoveries into clinical applications and elucidates clinical questions with the use of bench work, aiming to facilitate the prediction, prevention, diagnosis and treatment of diseases. The development of translational medicine will accelerate disease control and the process of finding solutions to key health problems. It is a multidisciplinary endeavor that integrates research from the medical sciences, basic sciences and social sciences, with the aim of optimizing patient care and preventive measures that may extend beyond health care services. Therefore, close and international collaboration between all parties involved is essential to the advancement of translational medicine. To enhance the aforementioned international collaboration as well as to provide a forum for communication and cross-pollenation between basic, translational and clinical research practitioners from all relevant established and emerging disciplines, the book series "Translational Medicine Research" features original and observational investigations in the broad fields of laboratory, clinical and public health research, aiming to provide practical and up-to-date information on significant research from all subspecialties of medicine and to broaden readers' vision horizons, from bench to bed and bed to bench.Produced in close collaboration with National Infrastructures for Translational Medicine (Shanghai), the largest translational medicine research center in China, the book series offers a state-of-the-art resource for physicians and researchers alike who are interested in the rapidly evolving field of translational medicine. Prof. Zhu Chen, the Editor-in-Chief of the series, is a hematologist at Shanghai Jiao Tong University, China's former Minister of Health, and chairman of the center's scientific advisory board.

More information about this series at http://www.springer.com/series/13024

Bin Ni · Xiang Guo · Qunfeng Guo
Editors

Atlantoaxial Fixation Techniques

Commonly Used and New Techniques

上海交通大學出版社
SHANGHAI JIAO TONG UNIVERSITY PRESS

Springer

Editors
Bin Ni
Department of Orthopedics
Changzheng Hospital
Shanghai
China

Xiang Guo
Department of Orthopedics
Changzheng Hospital
Shanghai
China

Qunfeng Guo
Department of Orthopedics
Changzheng Hospital
Shanghai
China

ISSN 2451-991X ISSN 2451-9928 (electronic)
Translational Medicine Research
ISBN 978-981-10-7888-0 ISBN 978-981-10-7889-7 (eBook)
https://doi.org/10.1007/978-981-10-7889-7

Library of Congress Control Number: 2018942237

Printed on acid-free paper

This Springer imprint is published by the registered company Springer Nature Singapore Pte Ltd.
part of Springer Nature
The registered company address is: 152 Beach Road, #21-01/04 Gateway East, Singapore 189721, Singapore

Preface

The development of internal spinal fixation has progressed rapidly, especially in regard to changes in occipital cervical fixation, from the earliest cable fixation technique to the present system of rod and screw fixation. The continuous upgrading of the system has made the operation more convenient and more effective. Although the traditional rod and screw fixation system can meet most surgical needs, the pursuit of a more complete fixation system to improve mechanical stability and meet the individual needs of the patient and the surgeon is still imperative for spinal surgeons. At present, innovations in the traditional internal fixation system are based on improvements of technique, combined with anatomical measurement and a biomechanical validation process. However, manufacturers of internal fixation devices are rarely involved in the development and promotion of improved instrumentation.

This book considers basic research methods in translational medicine as a guide, starting from clinical problems, linked with the clinical demand to improve fixation techniques through research in close collaboration with device manufacturers, leading to clinical trials and the marketing of internal fixation devices. The book focuses on a modified internal fixation technique for the upper cervical posterior approach, highlighting the trial of a reduction screw improvement, hook fixation, and anatomic line measurement of the pedicle screw arm, together with biomechanical validation, evaluation, and determination of the market demand for each part of the device. This book will clearly show the reader that the use of translational medicine in this context will aid in understanding the whole process of the modified posterior atlantoaxial internal fixation technique. In particular, through examples of translational medicine, the book will break through traditional thinking on the improvement of spinal fixation devices, advance translational medicine in regard to new ideas and specific operating procedures, and explain the best way to bring about improvements of spinal column fixation from the two aspects of theory and practice.

To improve spinal instrumentation is an important part of the spinal surgeon's research work. We believe that the new spinal instrumentation described in this book will be helpful for the majority of patients. We cordially recommend the book to the public, and devotedly hope that all readers can benefit from the book.

Shanghai, China Bin Ni
Shanghai, China Xiang Guo
Shanghai, China Qunfeng Guo

Contents

Part I
Introduction

Abstract

This section is an overview of the book. It firstly describes the regional anatomy and specific biomechanics of the atlantoaxial joint including bony, ligamentous, vascular and nerval anatomy, and the special biomechanical characters of atlantoaxial joint. The anatomic character of atlantoaxial joint can make reader better understand biomechanical character. Then, in the following chapter, the pathomechanics of atlantoaxial instability is elaborated. Many disorders, such as trauma, congenital and developmental anomalies, rheumatoid arthritis, degenerative disorders, inflammatory or infectious lesions, neoplasms, and secondary to some surgical intervention can lead to atlantoaxial instability. Early diagnosis and treatment are vital for patients. Therefore, in order to make proper diagnosis, the third chapter describes the common clinical symptoms and signs according to the cause, type, site, and specific situation of atlantoaxial instability. Meanwhile, the treatments of atlantoaxial instability (AAI), including non-surgical and surgical methods, are briefly reviewed and some modified atlantoaxial fixation techniques are introduced. Finally, some basic concepts of translation medicine which can effectively improve the translation from basic research to clinical application are stated.

Chapter 1
Applied Anatomy and Biomechanics of the Atlantoaxial Joint Complex

Bin Ni and Yuan Deng

Abstract Because of the special structure of atlantoaxial complex, there are a series of unique instrumentations for specific diseases in this important region. A thorough understanding of these relationships allows for a safe access to the cervical spine while minimizing complications. The first section of this chapter discusses the anatomy of the atlantoaxial joint complex, including bony, ligamentous, vascular, and nerval anatomy. The second section describes the outline of biomechanics of the atlantoaxial joint. The special biomechanical characters of the atlantoaxial joint arise from its unique anatomical construction. Therefore, appreciating the anatomical character of the atlantoaxial joint will provide the reader with a better understanding of its biomechanical character. Finally, the chapter describes several normal atlantoaxial fixation techniques, including anterior and posterior fixation, and motion-preserving devices.

1.1 Applied Anatomy of the Atlantoaxial Joint

1.1.1 Osseous Elements of the Atlantoaxial Complex

The ring-shaped atlas is the link of the occipital bone and axis, which is between occipital condyles and superior articular surfaces of axis (Fig. 1.1a, b). The posterior structure of the atlas, often called posterior arch, is a very important anatomy mark in atlantoaxial posterior approach surgery if it is complete which can have a rudimentary spinous process. But in up to 5% population, the posterior arch may be congenitally incomplete that should be paid with sufficient attention in posterior approach surgery in order to avoid iatrogenic spine injury [1].

B. Ni (✉)
Department of Orthopedics, Changzheng Hospital, Shanghai, China
e-mail: nibin99@sohu.com

Y. Deng
Department of Orthopedics, General Hospital of PLA, Beijing, China

B. Ni et al. (eds.), *Atlantoaxial Fixation Techniques*, Translational Medicine Research, https://doi.org/10.1007/978-981-10-7889-7_1

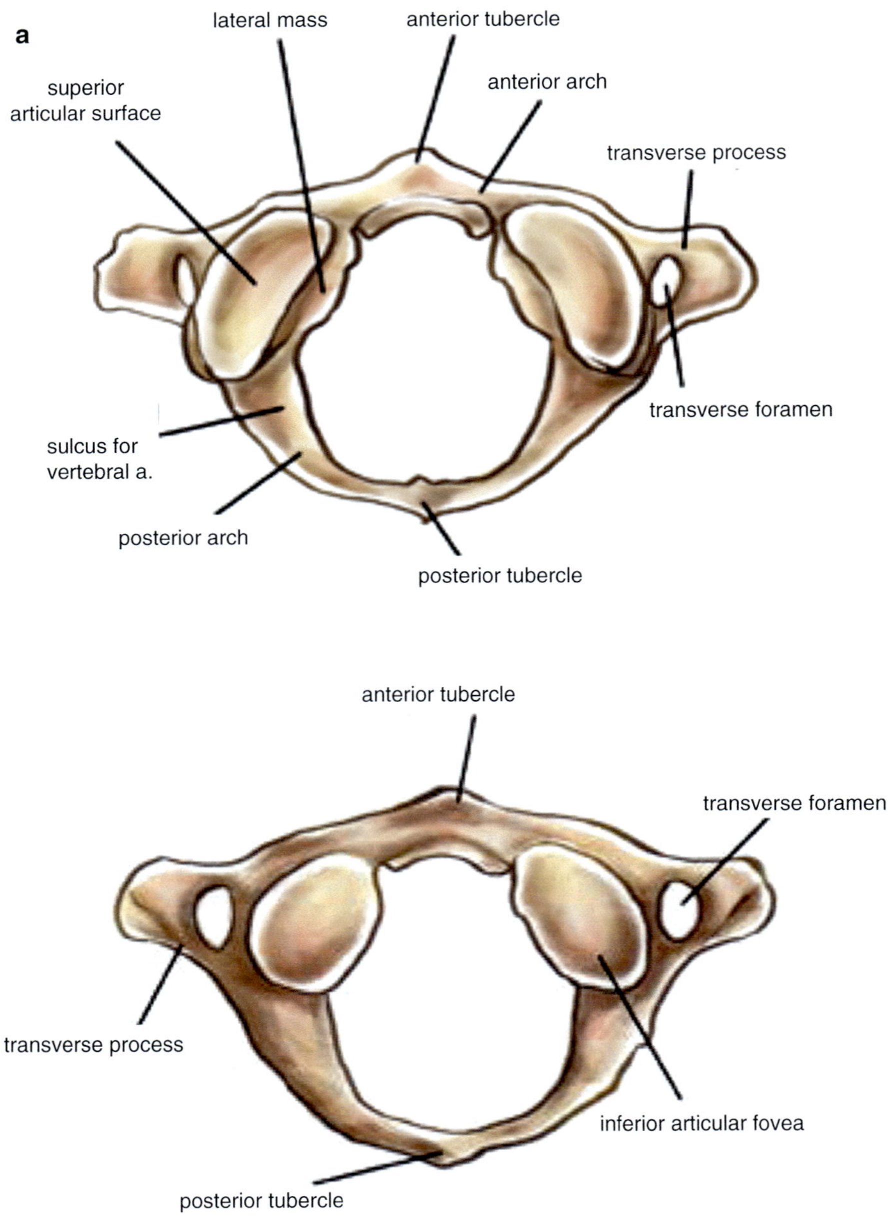

Fig. 1.1 (**a**) Atlas. (**b**) Axis

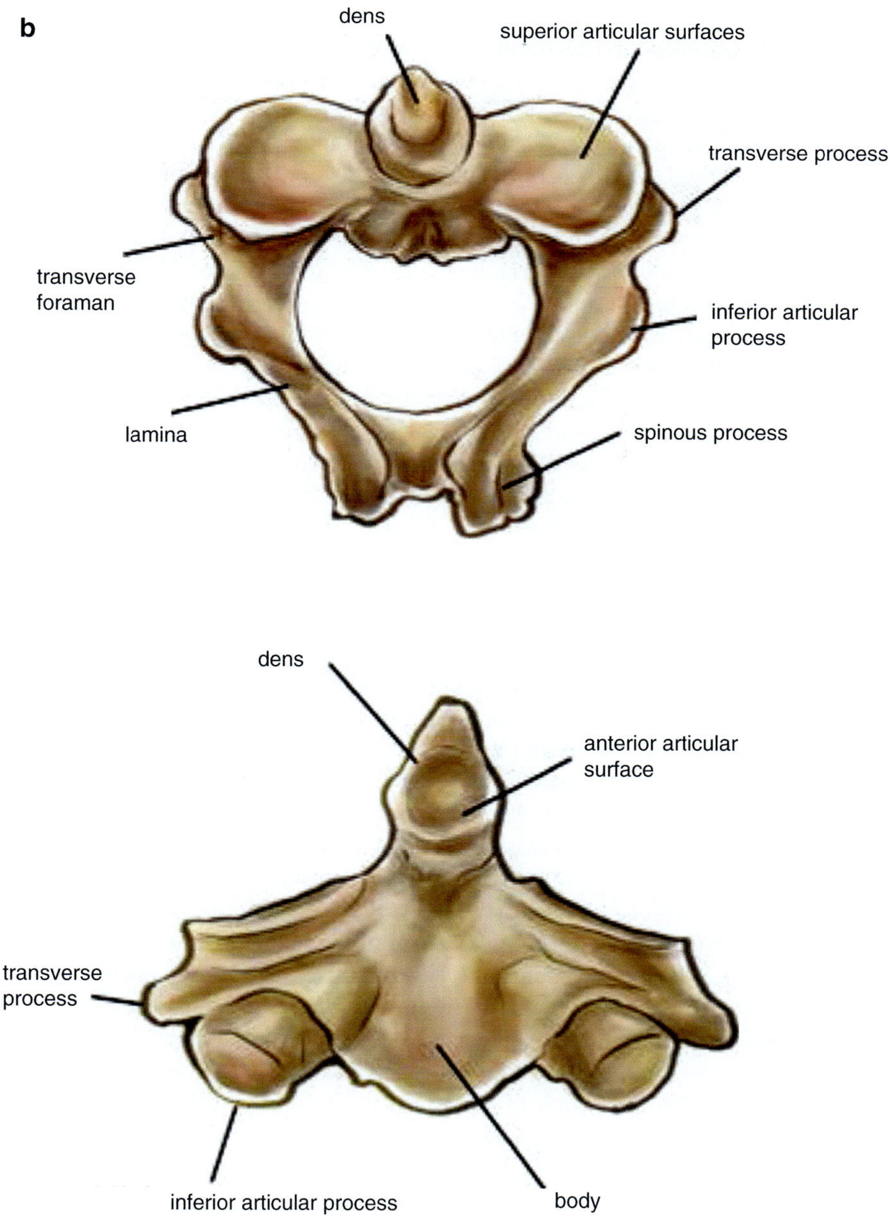

Fig. 1.1 (continued)

The anterior and medial bony structures of the atlas which is called the lateral mass are the position where the foramina transversaria localize. The vertebral artery which is located within the transverse process passes through the foramen transversarium and courses posteriorly within a sulcus on the superior aspect of the posterior arch of the atlas. An anomalous ossification, called the posterior ponticulus, which overlies the vertebral artery superiorly but appears to represent a widened C1 lamina and arch, may be seen in 12–19% of the general population. It may cause surgical implications when the clinical surgeon was going to identify anatomical landmarks for bony fixation of C1 [2–4]. The arch is fairly thin and sits closed to the odontoid process of the axis in anterior. The anterior tubercle of the atlas is the attachment point of the longus colli muscle and anterior longitudinal ligament, whereas the posterior tubercle serves as the bony attachments for the rectus minor muscle and suboccipital membrane. The average diameter of the spinal canal of the atlas is approximately 3 cm [5]. The angle between superior articular surfaces and horizontal surface is on average 129.4°, while the inferior articular surface angle is on average 130–135.8° [5, 6]. The atlanto-occipital articular surfaces allow comparable movement in flexion and extension [7–9]. The rotational mobility of atlanto-occipital joint is less than atlantoaxial joint because the shape of atlanto-occipital articular surface is slightly ellipsoid in nature and oblique.

To accommodate the specific anatomical structure of the atlas, many unique instrumentations are used. Although other techniques have been described recently that take better advantage of the specific anatomy of the region, the most popular way to fix the atlas is also by using sublaminar wiring. In posterior approach surgery, the lateral mass of the atlas can be an ideal place for screw placement [10–12]. To find the entry point of the lateral mass screw, identifying the C2 nerve root is the most important step before dissection. After exposing the C2 nerve root and the atlanto-axial articular, the entry point is most often below the overhanging arch in the middle of the exposed bone. The lateral screw should go through just above the joint with the anteromedial and cephalad trajectory in line with the shape of the lateral mass [10, 13]. Tan et al. reported that placing screws from the lamina of the lateral mass is acceptable [10], although the lamina of C1 is usually less than 5 mm thick [14].

The axis is also very special among cervical vertebrae. It is characterized by an odontoid process or dens that projects upward anteriorly, articulating with the posterior aspect of the anterior arch of the atlas as a synovial joint (Fig. 1.2a, b). Axial loads on the atlas tend to result in horizontal displacement of the lateral masses because of the unique bony configuration [15].

The dimensions of the dens are highly variable: Its mean height is 37.8 mm, its external transverse diameter is 9.3 mm, the internal transverse diameter is 4.5 mm, the mean anteroposterior external diameter is 10.5 mm, and the internal diameter is 6.2 mm [16]. The base of the dens is the narrowest portion, and the coronal and sagittal plane diameters are 8–10 mm and 10–11 mm, respectively [17, 18]. The articular between C2 and C3 is oblique apophyseal joint caudally, such as the subaxial cervical spine intervertebral joint. The bifid or partially bifid large spinous process is the first structure which can be seen during a posterior approach to the axis. In the posterior surgery, to identify the atlas, the C2 spinous process is a very

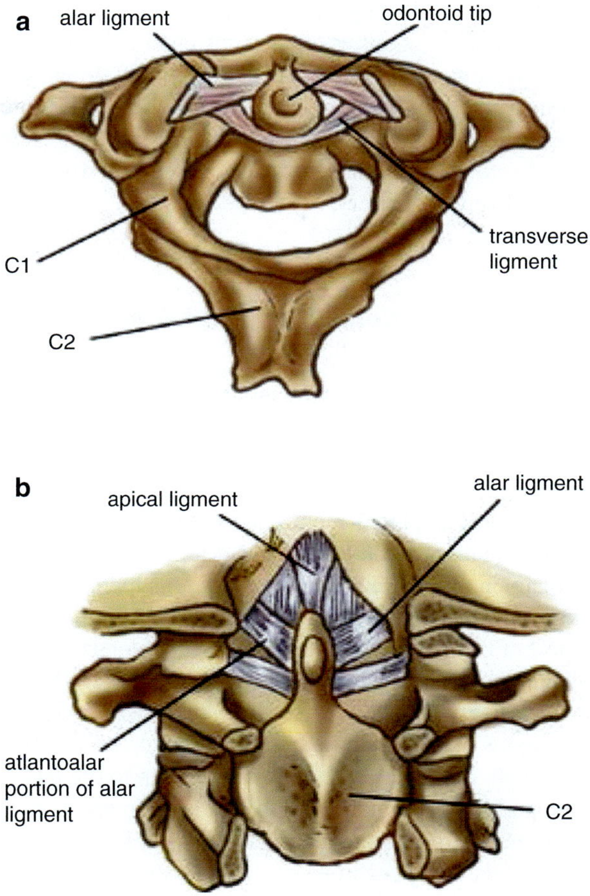

Fig. 1.2 (**a**, **b**) Atlantoaxial articulation and some related ligaments

important anatomy mark, because it often can be palpable through the skin. The large laminae of axis are different from any other subaxial cervical because of the big caudal and lateral inclination angle. There are two important structures at the junction of the lateral mass and lamina, pars interarticularis which is superiorly located on the junction and pedicle the medial portion of the pars (8 mm wide and 10 mm long) [19]. The pedicle of the axis is in a posterior-to-anterior direction that projects 30° medially and 20° superiorly [17]. The location of foramina transversaria of axis is somewhat variable in relation to lateral mass, pars interarticularis, and pedicles.

To consider the size of the C2 lateral mass, the standard screw is fitable. But there are still some other options that can be chosen because of the unique anatomy of this vertebra, for example, pars screw [20] and pedicle screw [21]. The screw through atlantoaxial articular usually passes the whole length of pars interarticularis from the inferior aspect of the lamina, and the end of the screw stops in the lateral mass of the atlas [22]. Because of the angle of the pars interarticularis and the favorable lie of the atlantoaxial joint the transarticular screw can be accessed, but more attention must be taken in surgical planning in order to identify the anatomy variability of the foramen transversarium and the vertebral artery. The absolute contraindication for using transarticular screw is the high risk of breaching vertebral artery during the procedure of screw placement that can be caused by a so-called "high-riding" or medially displaced vertebral artery.

1.1.2 Ligamentous Relationship of the Atlantoaxial Complex

In addition to the bony anatomy, the ligamentous attachments provide support to the cervical spine and associated articulations. In the atlanto-occipital complex, two membranous attachments, the anterior and posterior atlanto-occipital membranes, connect the anterior and posterior arch of C1 to the margins of the foramen magnum. The anterior atlanto-occipital membrane is the superior continuation of the anterior longitudinal ligament, whereas the posterior membrane is the superior continuation of the ligamentum flavum. The transverse ligament is the major stabilizer of the atlantoaxial complex (Fig. 1.2b). It attaches laterally to tubercles located on the posterior aspect of the anterior arch of C1, where it blends with the lateral mass. The length of the transverse ligament is 21.9 mm on average. Secondary stabilizers include the thick alar ligament, which arises from the sides of the dens to the medial aspects of the condyles of the occipital bone at an angle of 140–180° [7], and the apical ligament, which arises from the apex of the dens to the anterior edge of the foramen magnum and has an average length of 23.5 mm and a 20-degree anterior tilt [23]. The transverse ligament and alar ligaments stabilize this atlantoaxial complex; however, in the face of ligamentous laxity or disruption, the joint is ill equipped to handle the required multiaxial movements. In some individuals, an anterior atlantodental ligament exists connecting the base of the dens to the anterior arch of the atlas [24]. The tectorial membrane, the superior continuation of the posterior longitudinal ligament, covers the dens and all the occipitoaxial ligaments and extends from the posterior body of C2 to the basilar portion of the occipital bone and the anterior aspect of the foramen magnum.

1.1.3 Vascular Anatomy of the Atlantoaxial Complex

Although the vertebral artery takes a relatively straight course through the transverse foramina of C6 through C3, the change of direction just above the transverse foramen of C2 must be focused by the clinical surgeon (Fig. 1.3).

When the vertebral artery exits the foramen transversarium of C2, it is no longer covered dorsally by the bone. The vertebral artery takes a special pathway at the atlantoaxial region. It first goes laterally, then enters the foramen transversarium of

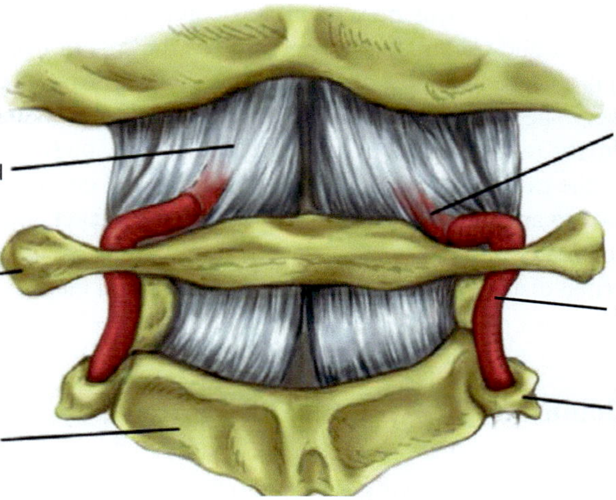

Fig. 1.3 C1–2 level of vertebral artery

the atlas, and after that bends posteromedially dorsal to the lateral mass of the atlas. The artery turns cranially to go through the foramen magnum via the dura. The surgeon will have some difficulties during decompression and instrumentation by virtue of the anatomical variation of the vertebral artery and branches. As mentioned above, the posterior ponticulus may appear falsely as a widened C1 arch [2–4]. The persistent intersegmental artery is another important anatomical variant, which may occupy the space of C2 nerve root that should be cared during the posterior approach surgery. Four percent of the general population may have it unilaterally and less than 1% may have it bilaterally [4, 25, 26]. There are some rare but real anatomical variants in atlantoaxial region like a fenestrated segment of the vertebral artery and a takeoff of the posteroinferior cerebellar artery [4, 26].

1.1.4 Nerve Distribution of the Atlantoaxial Complex

The first cervical nerve, or suboccipital nerve, exits the vertebral canal above the posterior arch of the atlas and posteromedial to the lateral mass, lying between the vertebral artery and the posterior arch. The posterior primary ramus of the first cervical nerve enters the suboccipital triangle and sends motor fibers to the deep muscles. The anterior primary ramus of the first cervical nerve forms a loop with the second anterior primary ramus and sends fibers to the hypoglossal nerve. The cervical plexus receives fibers from anterior primary rami of C1–4. The cervical plexus is located opposite C1–3, ventral and lateral to the levator scapulae and middle scalene muscles. The cervical plexus has distributions to the skin and muscles, such as the rectus capitis anterior and lateralis, longus capitis and cervicis, levator scapulae, and middle scalene. The cervical plexus forms loops and branches to supply the sternocleidomastoid and trapezius muscles. It has communications with the hypoglossal nerve from C1 and C2 and leaves this trunk as the superior root of the ansa cervicalis, which is a nerve loop formed with the inferior root from C2 and C3. The second cervical nerve lies on the lamina of the axis, posterior to the lateral mass, and the posterior primary ramus, or the greater occipital nerve, pierces the trapezius about 2 cm below the external occipital protuberance and 2–4 cm from the midline. Trauma or irritation to any of the three terminal nerves (the greater and lesser occipital nerve and the greater auricular nerve) can produce pain, headache, or hyperesthesia in their dermal distribution over the occiput and around the ear.

1.2 Biomechanics of the Atlantoaxial Joint

The upper cervical spine consists of the occiput (C0), the atlas (C1), and the axis (C2). The unique anatomy of this region leads to complex biomechanical behavior. It has more axial rotation than any other regions in the entire spine. The axial rotation of the atlantoaxial motion segment can reach 80° [27]. The flexion extension range of motion at C12 can reach 20–30° [27]. This range of motion is similar to that of C01. Lateral bending at the atlantoaxial joint is similar to that of the lower cervical spine, with an average motion of 7–8°.

The atlantoaxial joint complex has many ligaments, such as anterior longitudinal ligament, apical ligament, alar ligaments, cruciate ligament, tectorial membrane ligament, and posterior atlantoaxial ligament. There is no cervical disc between C1 and C2. The large motion is attributed to the articulating joints, along with numerous ligaments attached to various locations on the vertebrae. The transverse ligament (or the lateral bands of the cruciate ligament) is probably the most important structure of the upper cervical spine and restrains C1/2 motion in almost all directions [28]. It also prevents C1 from excessive anterior translation. Unfortunately, this ligament is susceptible to injury from external impact forces. The alar ligaments insert symmetrically on the dens, with one portion attached to the occiput and the other attached to the atlas. The alar ligaments restrict axial rotation, although its range of motion is large [29]. The vertical band of the cruciate ligament was shown to stabilize the atlantoaxial joint in lateral bending [28]. However, this result has not been confirmed in other studies. Panjabi suggested that the lateral bending motion was primarily restrained by the alar ligaments [27]. The atlantoaxial joint does not have tight joint capsules and allows large motion in axial rotation. It also has weak support in lateral bending and flexion extension. However, the joint offers gliding surfaces in various loading directions.

Like the lower cervical spine, the upper cervical spine has coupled motion. Coupled motion refers to the motion in which the rotation of a vertebra along a certain axis is associated with simultaneous rotation or translation in other axes. Early studies only reported coupled vertical translation of C1 in an axial rotation [27]. A recent in vitro study suggested that coupled motion occurred in all three loading directions: flexion extension (FE), lateral bending, and axial rotation. For example, 10 degrees of FE motion at C12 introduced 2.6 and 14.4° in lateral bending and axial rotation, respectively. The lateral bending motion of 4.1° induced 3.7 and 18.3° in flexion extension and axial rotation, respectively. A large axial rotation of 68° also led to significant motion in flexion extension (11.7°) and lateral bending (11.7°). These results suggested that coupled motion was significant at the atlantoaxial joint in all loading directions.

A large number of fixation options have been proposed for atlantoaxial joint instability. In 1939, Gallie used posterior wiring and bone grafts to treat atlantoaxial instability. This technique is a one-point fixation and has poor fixation strength. In the late 1980s, Magerl and Seeman introduced a transarticular screw fixation technique combined with posterior wiring. This technique provides three-point fixation and offers exceptional construct stability. However, it is technically demanding, and there are a significant portion of patients whose anatomy may not allow such screw trajectory. Without posterior wiring, this technique has reduced fixation strength in flexion extension [30]. Since then, other treatment options have also been proposed. Harms introduced posterior fixation with C1 lateral mass screws and C2 pedicle screws connected with titanium rods [31]. This technique is easier to apply with modern polyaxial screws. Its construct rigidity is comparable to that of the traditional Magerl technique or C12 transarticular screws [32]. The C1 claw is a novel device that connects the C1 posterior arch to C2 pedicle screws with rods. This configuration offers adequate fixation strength. The claw can also be used with C2 laminar hooks; however, this option has less construct stability [30]. Anatomy permitting, bilateral C1 claws combined with transarticular screws offer the highest construct stability [12]. Alternatively, C1 lateral mass screws can be connected to C2 intralaminar screws. This surgical option may be useful in some cases, because C2 intralaminar screws are easier to place. However, they appear to have weaker strength unless a cross-link is added to the construct [33].

Goel proposed C1/2 joint spacers to facilitate vertical reduction of basilar invagination [34]. The bilateral joint spacers provide additional load-bearing surfaces and are particularly useful when the upper cervical becomes unstable. Biomechanical data suggested that this technique offered exceptional construct stability [35, 36]. However, it must also be recognized that this technique might sacrifice the C2 nerves, especially in patients with complex C12 deformities. To avoid vertebral artery injury, a modification of this technique is the integrated C12 spacers, which accommodate screws for the C1 lateral mass and C2 lamina. Its biomechanical strength was shown to be comparable to that of the Harms technique [37].

In addition to the posterior fixation techniques, several anterior surgical options have been proposed [38–40]. C1/2 anterior transarticular screws were shown to have acceptable construct stability [38]. However, the C12 anterior Harms plate/screw system did not seem to offer adequate fixation strength [38]. Another choice is the transoral atlantoaxial reduction plate (TARP) [39, 40]. The TARP is an "n"-shaped plate that completes the anterior ring of the atlas. It has four holes on the plate corners to fit four screws, two for each vertebra. Combined with C12 joint spacers, this technique has exceptional construct rigidity. Finite element analysis showed that it had better fixation strength than the posterior Goel technique [41].

A more recent novel device is the integrated C1/2 joint spacer, which includes two screws inserted onto C1 and C2, respectively [42]. This device has an ultralow profile and can be used to avoid dysphagia. Although its biomechanical strength is lower than that of the TARP [43], early clinical results suggested that this was a safe and effective treatment option [42].

Motion-preserving devices have also been developed in recent years [44, 45]. The objective of these devices is to mimic the physiological motion of the atlanto-axial joint in all three directions. Although such devices could reproduce normal C1/2 motion in cadaveric models [45], the long-term clinical efficacy of these devices has yet to be confirmed.

References

1. Gehweiler JA Jr, Daffner RH, Roberts L Jr. Malformations of the atlas vertebra simulating the Jefferson fracture. AJR Am J Roentgenol. 1983;140:1083–6.
2. Hasan M, Shukla S, Siddiqui MS, et al. Posterolateral tunnels and ponticuli in human atlas vertebrae. J Anat. 2001;199:339–43.
3. Young JP, Young PH, Ackermann MJ, et al. The ponticulus posticus: implications for screw insertion into the first cervical lateral mass. J Bone Joint Surg Am. 2005;87:2495–8.
4. Hong JT, Lee SW, Son BC, et al. Analysis of anatomical variations of bone and vascular structures around the posterior atlantal arch using three-dimensional computed tomography angiography. J Neurosurg Spine. 2008;8:230–6.
5. Konig SA, Goldammer A, Vitzthum HE. Anatomical data on the craniocervical junction and their correlation with degenerative changes in 30 cadaveric specimens. J Neurosurg Spine. 2005;3:379–85.
6. Cattrysse E, Provyn S, Gagey O, et al. In vitro three dimensional morphometry of the lateral atlantoaxial articular surfaces. Spine (Phila PA 1976). 2008;33:1503–8.
7. Panjabi M, Dvorak J, Crisco JJ 3rd, et al. Effects of alar ligament transection on upper cervical spine rotation. J Orthop Res. 1991;9:584–93.
8. Panjabi M, Dvorak J, Crisco J 3rd, et al. Flexion, extension, and lateral bending of the upper cervical spine in response to alar ligament transections. J Spinal Disord. 1991;4:157–67.
9. Zhang H, Bai J. Development and validation of a finite element model of the occipito-atlantoaxial complex under physiologic loads. Spine (Phila PA 1976). 2007;32:968–74.
10. Tan M, Wang H, Wang Y, et al. Morphometric evaluation of screw fixation in atlas via posterior arch and lateral mass. Spine (Phila PA 1976). 2003;28:888–95.
11. Dong Y, Hong MX, Jianyi L, et al. Quantitative anatomy of the lateral mass of the atlas. Spine (Phila PA 1976). 2003;28:860–3.
12. Richter M, Schmidt R, Claes L, et al. Posterior atlantoaxial fixation: biomechanical in vitro comparison of six different techniques. Spine (Phila PA 1976). 2002;27:1724–32.
13. Ahmed R, Traynelis VC, Menezes AH. Fusions at the craniovertebral junction. Childs Nerv Syst. 2008;24:1209–24.
14. Lee MJ, Cassinelli E, Riew KD. The feasibility of inserting atlas lateral mass screws via the posterior arch. Spine (Phila PA 1976). 2006;31:2798–801.
15. Hays MB, Alker GJ Jr. Fractures of the atlas vertebra. The two-part burst fracture of Jefferson. Spine (Phila PA 1976). 1988;13:601–3.
16. Heller JG, Alson MD, Schaffler MB, et al. Quantitative internal dens morphology. Spine (Phila PA 1976). 1992;17:861–6.
17. Xu R, Nadaud MC, Ebraheim NA, et al. Morphology of the second cervical vertebra and the posterior projection of the C2 pedicle axis. Spine (Phila PA 1976). 1995;20:259–63.

18. Schaffler MB, Alson MD, Heller JG, et al. Morphology of the dens. A quantitative study. Spine (Phila PA 1976). 1992;17:738–43.
19. An HS, Gordin R, Renner K. Anatomic considerations for plate-screw fixation of the cervical spine. Spine (Phila PA 1976). 1991;16:S548–51.
20. Wellman BJ, Follett KA, Traynelis VC. Complications of posterior articular mass plate fixation of the subaxial cervical spine in 43 consecutive patients. Spine (Phila PA 1976). 1998;23:193–200.
21. Borne GM, Bedou GL, Pinaudeau M. Treatment of pedicular fractures of the axis. A clinical study and screw fixation technique. J Neurosurg. 1984;60:88–93.
22. Magerl F, Seemann PS. Stable posterior fusion of the atlas and axis by transarticular screw fixation. In: Cervical spine. Vienna: Springer; 1987. p. 217–21.
23. Panjabi MM, Oxland TR, Parks EH. Quantitative anatomy of cervical spine ligaments. Part I. Upper cervical spine. J Spinal Disord. 1991;4:270–6.
24. Dvorak J, Panjabi MM. Functional anatomy of the alar ligaments. Spine (Phila PA 1976). 1987;12:183–9.
25. Sato K, Watanabe T, Yoshimoto T, et al. Magnetic resonance imaging of C2 segmental type of vertebral artery. Surg Neurol. 1994;41:45–51.
26. Tokuda K, Miyasaka K, Abe H, et al. Anomalous atlantoaxial portions of vertebral and posterior inferior cerebellar arteries. Neuroradiology. 1985;27:410–3.
27. White AA, Panjabi MM. Kinematics of the spine. In: Clinical biomechanics of the spine. 2nd ed. Philadelphia: J.B. Lippincott; 1990. p. 85–120.
28. Radcliff KE, Hussain MM, Moldavsky M, et al. In vitro biomechanics of the craniocervical junction-a sequential sectioning of its stabilizing structures. Spine J. 2015;15:1618–28.
29. Dvorak J, Schneider E, Saldinger P, et al. Biomechanics of the craniocervical region: the alar and transverse ligaments. J Orthop Res. 1988;6:452–61.
30. Henriques T, Cunningham BW, Olerud C, et al. Biomechanical comparison of five different atlantoaxial posterior fixation techniques. Spine (Phila PA 1976). 2000;25:2877–83.
31. Harms J, Melcher RP. Posterior C1-C2 fusion with polyaxial screw and rod fixation. Spine (Phila PA 1976). 2001;26:2467–71.
32. Puttlitz CM, Melcher RP, Kleinstueck FS, et al. Stability analysis of craniovertebral junction fixation techniques. J Bone Joint Surg Am. 2004;86-A:561–8.
33. Lehman RA Jr, Dmitriev AE, Wilson KW. Biomechanical analysis of the C2 intralaminar fixation technique using a cross-link and offset connector for an unstable atlantoaxial joint. Spine J. 2012;12:151–6.
34. Goel A, Kulkarni AG, Sharma P. Reduction of fixed atlantoaxial dislocation in 24 cases: technical note. J Neurosurg Spine. 2005;2:505–9.
35. Li S, Ni B, Xie N, et al. Biomechanical evaluation of an atlantoaxial lateral mass fusion cage with C1-C2 pedicle fixation. Spine (Phila PA 1976). 2010;35:E624–32.
36. Park J, Scheer JK, Lim TJ, et al. Biomechanical analysis of Goel technique for C1-2 fusion. J Neurosurg Spine. 2011;14:639–46.
37. Robertson PA, Tsitsopoulos PP, Voronov LI, et al. Biomechanical investigation of a novel integrated device for intra-articular stabilization of the C1-C2 (atlantoaxial) joint. Spine J. 2012;12:136–42.
38. Kim SM, Lim TJ, Paterno J, et al. Biomechanical comparison of anterior and posterior stabilization methods in atlantoaxial instability. J Neurosurg. 2004;100:277–83.
39. Ai FZ, Yin QS, DC X, et al. Transoral atlantoaxial reduction plate internal fixation with transoral transpedicular or articular mass screw of c2 for the treatment of irreducible atlantoaxial dislocation: two case reports. Spine (Phila PA 1976). 2011;36:E556–62.
40. Xia H, Yin Q, Ai F, et al. Treatment of basilar invagination with atlantoaxial dislocation: atlantoaxial joint distraction and fixation with transoral atlantoaxial reduction plate (TARP) without odontoidectomy. Eur Spine J. 2014;23:1648–55.
41. Zhang B, Liu H, Cai X, et al. Biomechanical comparison of modified TARP technique versus modified goel technique for the treatment of basilar invagination: a finite element analysis. Spine (Phila PA 1976). 2016;41:E459–66.

42. Kasliwal MK, O'Toole JE. Integrated intervertebral device for anterior cervical fusion: an initial experience. J Craniovertebr Junction Spine. 2012;3:52–7.
43. Zhang BC, Liu HB, Cai XH, et al. Biomechanical comparison of a novel transoral atlantoaxial anchored cage with established fixation technique – a finite element analysis. BMC Musculoskelet Disord. 2015;16:261.
44. Hu Y, YJ G, He XF, et al. Biomechanical evaluation of stability and three-dimensional movements of the atlantoaxial joint after artificial atlanto-odontoid joint arthroplasty. Orthop Surg. 2010;2:111–8.
45. Kato K, Yokoyama T, Ono A, et al. Novel motion preservation device for atlantoaxial instability. J Spinal Disord Tech. 2013;26:E107–11.

Chapter 2
Pathomechanics of Atlantoaxial Instability

Chunhui Wu and Xuhui Zhou

Abstract Atlantoaxial instability can arise from different disorders, including trauma, congenital and developmental anomalies, rheumatoid arthritis, degenerative disorders, inflammatory or infectious lesions, neoplasms, and secondary to certain surgical interventions. This chapter describes the pathomechanics of atlantoaxial instability resulting from atlas and axis fractures, congenital and developmental abnormalities, and rheumatoid arthritis.

The craniovertebral junction, as a bridge connecting the skull to the spine, which is adjacent to the high-level spinal cord, vertebra arteries, and other important anatomical structures, consists mainly of the foramen magnum, the atlas, and the axis. Most axial rotatory motion and some flexion-extension and lateral bending motion of the normal cervical spine occur in the craniovertebral junction. Thus, it is of vital importance to be adapted for stability and motion. The atlantoaxial joint, the most mobile part of the craniovertebral junction, is responsible for nearly 50% of rotatory motion, about 40° on each side [1, 2]. Clinical atlantoaxial instability indicates that some hypermotion or abnormal movement exists between the atlas and the axis under physiological load, which might lead to clinical problems of pain and neurological damage.

From an anatomical perspective, in contrast to that of the atlanto-occipital joint, the articular surfaces of C1 and C2 are both convex rather than ball and socket, and they are surrounded by a looser joint capsule, allowing more freedom of motion. Thus, atlantoaxial stability is attributed to the intactness of the bony and ligamentous structures.

There are many anatomical structures that affect the stability of C1–C2, such as transverse ligaments, dentate ligaments, the apical and alar ligaments, and the joint capsules. The dentate, alar, and apical ligaments are considered secondary

C. Wu (✉)
Weigao Orthopedic Device Co., Ltd, Weihai, China
e-mail: 1921379577@qq.com

X. Zhou
Department of Orthopedics, Changzheng Hospital, Shanghai, China

B. Ni et al. (eds.), *Atlantoaxial Fixation Techniques*, Translational Medicine Research, https://doi.org/10.1007/978-981-10-7889-7_2

stabilizers of C1–C2. The cruciate ligament, the most pivotal portion of which is the transverse ligament, is the major stabilizer. During head flexion, the transverse ligament provides restriction to the anterior translation of the atlas and permits the rotation movement around the dens. The odontoid articulates with the anterior arch of the C1 ring and provides translational restraint against horizontal displacement of the atlas of the axis, acting as a pivot, about which the atlas rotates. Thus, atlantoaxial instability can arise from many different disorders, including trauma, congenital and developmental anomalies, rheumatoid arthritis, degenerative disorders, inflammatory or infectious lesions, neoplasms, and secondary to certain surgical interventions.

2.1 Atlas and Axis Fractures

Type II or III atlas fractures (involving the equator of the atlas having two and more fractures or involving the lateral mass) [3] usually combine with transverse ligament injury, which was described by Spence [4] (summarized as a C1 lateral mass overhang of more than 6.9 mm in an open position X-ray film). Type II odontoid process fractures are classified according to Anderson and D'Alonzo [5] and are common conditions leading to atlantoaxial instability.

2.2 Congenital and Developmental Abnormalities

Failure in the development and correct connection of the atlas and axis that occurs before birth is referred to as a congenital anomaly, for example, basilar invagination, atlas assimilation, and odontoid aplasia. Developmental abnormalities are those that occur postnatally during the period of unfinished bone growth, including basilar impression, os odontoideum, and other syndromal abnormalities [6]. Os odontoideum is a corticated smooth oval or round ossicle at the tip of the odontoid process that has no osseous continuity with the body of C2.

2.3 Rheumatoid Arthritis

Rheumatoid arthritis (RA) is the most common inflammatory disease of the cervical spine, and 20–86% of RA patients have atlantoaxial instability [7–9]. RA-associated inflammatory synovitis erodes the joint cavities, cartilage, local bone, and associated ligaments, leading to atlantoaxial instability.

References

1. Monckeberg JE, Tome CV, Matias A, et al. CT scan study of atlantoaxial rotatory mobility in asymptomatic adult subjects: a basis for better understanding C1-C2 rotatory fixation and subluxation. Spine (Phila PA 1976). 2009;34:1292–5.
2. White APM. Kinematics of the spine. Philadelphia: Lippincott; 1990.
3. Landells CD, Van Peteghem PK. Fractures of the atlas: classification, treatment and morbidity. Spine (Phila PA 1976). 1988;13:450–2.
4. Spence KF Jr, Decker S, Sell KW. Bursting atlantal fracture associated with rupture of the transverse ligament. J Bone Joint Surg Am. 1970;52:543–9.
5. Anderson LD, D'Alonzo RT. Fractures of the odontoid process of the axis. J Bone Joint Surg Am. 1974;56:1663–74.
6. Menezes AH. Craniocervical developmental anatomy and its implications. Childs Nerv Syst. 2008;24:1109–22.
7. Dreyer SJ, Boden SD. Natural history of rheumatoid arthritis of the cervical spine. Clin Orthop Relat Res. 1999;366:98–106.
8. Casey AT, Crockard HA, Pringle J, O'Brien MF, Stevens JM. Rheumatoid arthritis of the cervical spine: current techniques for management. Orthop Clin North Am. 2002;33(2):291–309.
9. Nguyen HV, Ludwig SC, Silber J, et al. Rheumatoid arthritis of the cervical spine. Spine J. 2004;4(3):329–34.

Chapter 3
Diagnosis and Treatment of Atlantoaxial Instability

Jeffrey Scott Fischgrund and Jian Yang

Abstract Atlantoaxial instability (AAI) is characterized by excessive movement at the junction between the atlas (C1) and the axis (C2), as a result of either a bony or ligamentous abnormality. Early diagnosis and treatment are vital for patients. Clinical symptoms and signs may be different according to the cause, type, site, and specific situation of the atlantoaxial instability. Neurological dysfunction can occur when the spinal cord or adjacent nerve roots are involved. Imaging examinations, especially computed tomography and magnetic resonance imaging (MRI), can provide visual evidence to make a proper diagnosis. Treatments for AAI can be nonsurgical or surgical. The nonsurgical treatments include relative pharmacotherapy and routine immobilization methods. Surgical treatments comprise treatment of primary upper cervical diseases and/or trauma and techniques of C1–C2 fusion (C1–C2 fusion is discussed briefly because it is covered in depth in the following chapter).

3.1 Symptoms of Atlantoaxial Instability

Clinical symptoms can differ according to the cause, type, site, and specific situation of AAI. Patients with longer duration of the disease have relatively mild clinical manifestations, while those of patients with acute exacerbation are more serious. AAI that results from trauma can lead to high-level spinal cord injury (SCI), which affects the respiratory and cardiovascular center seriously, even becoming life threatening.

Pediatric patients, whose spinal canal volume is somewhat larger than that of adult patients' because of immature spinal development, occasionally show no obvious clinical symptoms or signs because of the sufficient space available for the spinal cord (SAC) (Figs. 3.1 and 3.2). In clinical practice, some patients with AAI

J. S. Fischgrund (✉)
Department of Orthopaedic Surgery, William Beaumont Hospital, Royal Oak, MI, USA

J. Yang
Department of Orthopedics, Qingdao Municipal Hospital, Qingdao, China

B. Ni et al. (eds.), *Atlantoaxial Fixation Techniques*, Translational Medicine Research, https://doi.org/10.1007/978-981-10-7889-7_3

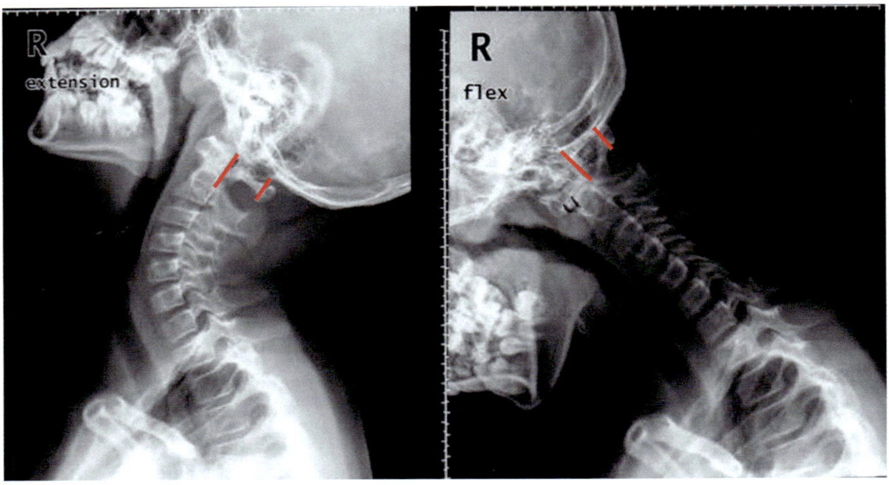

Fig. 3.1 Sufficient SAC in pediatric patients

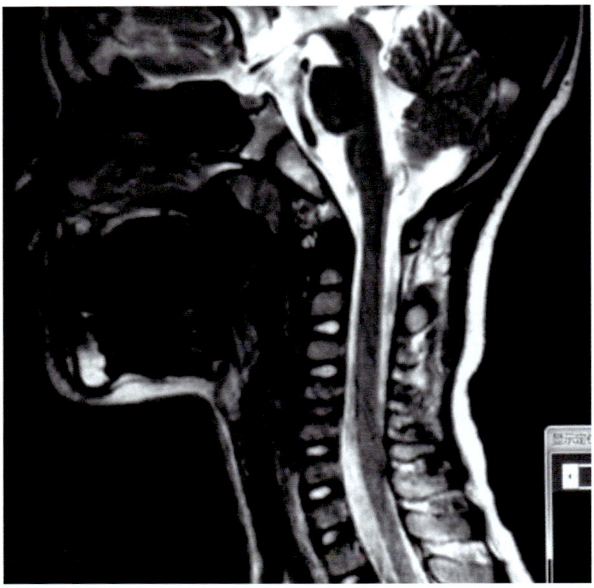

Fig. 3.2 The spinal canal volume is sufficient for the spinal cord

only suffer local occipital and occipitocervical pain, without neurological dysfunction. Most AAI patients' first symptoms are pain at the back of the head caused by compression of the major occipital nerve, followed by numbness or loss of strength of all four limbs; however, other patients might complain of torticollis on initial presentation (Fig. 3.3). Most patients with AAI will suffer varying degrees of

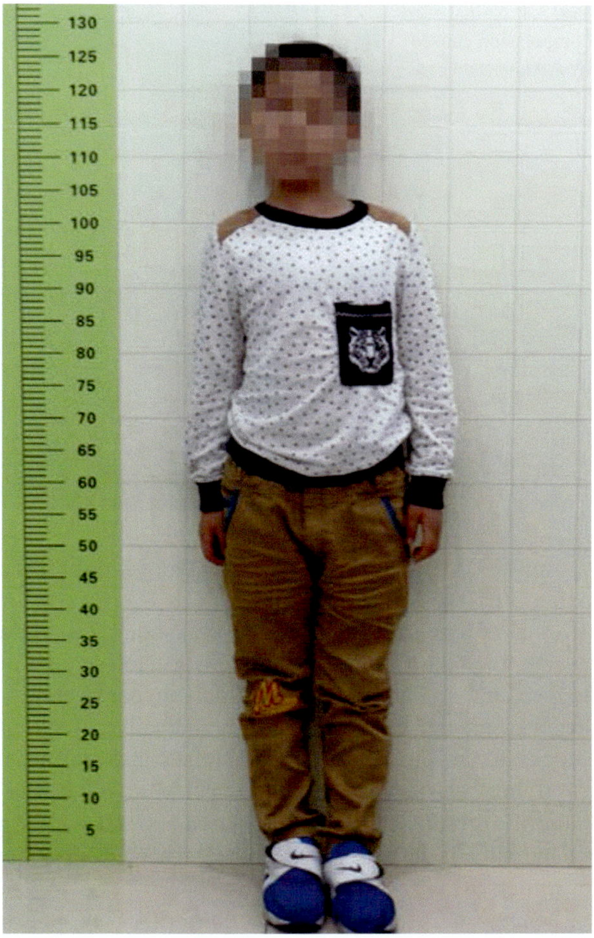

Fig. 3.3 Torticollis caused by AAI

restricted cervical movement; in particular, the degree of cervical rotational activity could be reduced by more than 50%.

3.2 Signs of Atlantoaxial Instability

Neurological dysfunction can be caused by spinal cord compression resulting from the displacement between the atlas and axis (Fig. 3.4). Occasionally, spinal cord compression can arise or worsen if susceptible patients are subjected to extreme ranges of motion. Progressive neurological dysfunction can include upper motor neuron signs, such as spasticity, myelopathy, and radicular signs, which produce

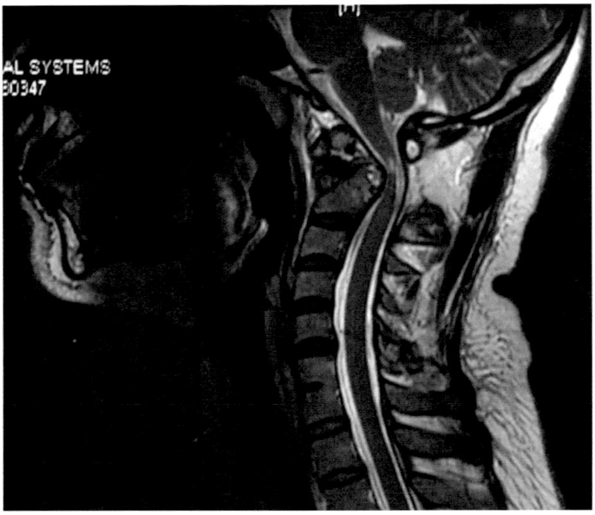

Fig. 3.4 Spinal cord compression caused by AAI

symptoms that include dystonia, walking instability, numbness of all four limbs, and muscle weakness.

A careful neurological examination should be conducted, especially for patients at risk, including assessment of sensory, motor, and other neurological functions. Upper motor neuron signs, including hypermyotonia, hyperreflexia, clonus, and extensor plantar reflexes, might be indicative of symptomatic AAI. A somatosensory evoked response might reveal information regarding neurological involvement. A "drunk" or staggering gait, decreased myodynamia of all four limbs, and even muscular atrophy can also be found in patients with symptomatic AAI.

Individuals with rotatory displacement often present with a cock-robin deformity or torticollis.

Many patients with rheumatoid arthritis (RA) present with occipital tenderness. Others develop myelopathy, vertigo, brainstem signs, or lower cranial nerve palsies. The brainstem findings show either basilar invaginations or the alteration of the path of the vertebral artery with a change in the normal anatomy. Rana reported the subtle association of the involvement of the fifth cranial nerve, which has a descending tract that extends to C2. Pyramidal signs, including hyperactive reflexes, positive Hoffmann sign, positive Babinski sign, and proprioceptive loss, should alert the physician to developing myelopathy.

AAI patients with Arnold-Chiari malformation (a malformation of the brain that comprises of a downward displacement of the cerebellar tonsils and the medulla oblongata through the foramen magnum) can present with cerebellar dysfunction, such as ataxia. AAI with Arnold-Chiari malformation can also cause hydrocephalus as a result of obstruction of the outflow of cerebrospinal fluid.

The most specific physical findings in patients with symptomatic AAI secondary to infections of the head and neck are torticollis, tenderness over the spinous process of the axis with palpation, and the Sudeck sign (displacement of the axis of the

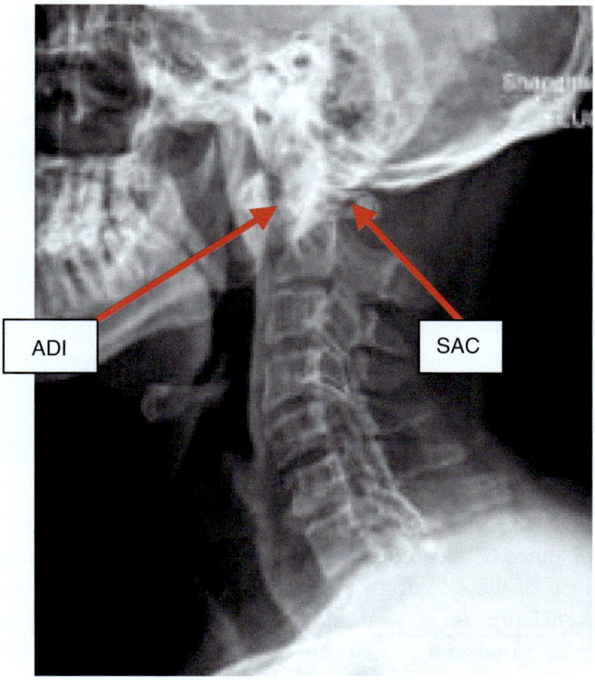

Fig. 3.5 ADI and SAC

spine in the direction of head tilt). A reduction in size of the nasopharynx and increased nasal resonance may also be presented because of the forward displacement of the anterior arch of the atlas. Patients with atlantoaxial subluxation (AAS) caused by inflammatory processes exhibit signs of root or cord involvement less frequently.

3.3 Imaging Exams

3.3.1 Plain Radiography

Plain radiography has been the primary means of imaging the cervical spine. This method is inexpensive, reliable, and widely available. Newer techniques, such as computed tomography (CT) and MRI, have advanced the way we image the spine but do not substitute for the information provided by a plain X-ray.

Lateral, anteroposterior, and open-mouth views represent the routine radiographic evaluation of the cervical spine. The lateral view is a critical part of the radiographic evaluation of the cervical spine. A lateral X-ray must include the base of the skull to the cervicothoracic junction. The anterior atlantodens interval (AADI or ADI) should be evaluated for excess widening (Fig. 3.5). The AADI or ADI has

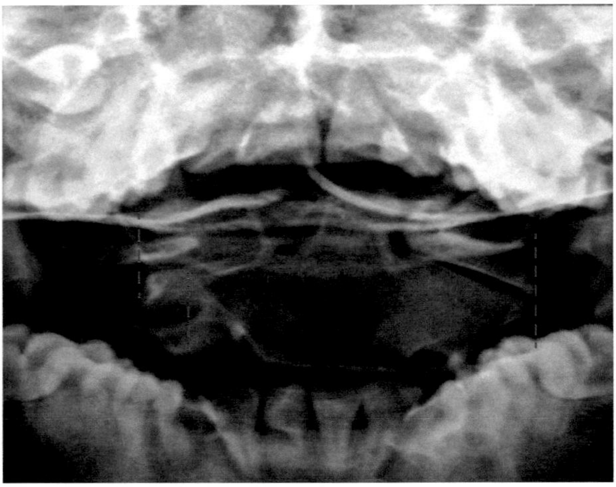

Fig. 3.6 Open-mouth X-ray of C1–C2 articulation. The line represents the lateral masses of C1 and C2

been used traditionally as a measure of atlantoaxial instability. The AADI is the distance between the posterior edge of the anterior ring of C1 and the anterior surface of the odontoid process. In adults, the AADI should be less than 3.5 mm of translation on flexion and extension views [1]. This measurement should be less than 5 mm in a pediatric patient [2]. It is important to note that these values were obtained from evaluation of normal cervical spines. These values may not be applicable to specific disease states. An example of this is the case with Down syndrome, where larger values may be considered normal. It has been suggested that the posterior atlantodens interval (PADI) might be more useful to identify patients at risk of neurological compromise. The PADI is the distance between the posterior border of the odontoid process and the anterior margin of the posterior ring of C1. This measure is a reflection of the SAC (Fig. 3.5). Boden et al. [3] found that the PADI correlated with severity of neurological symptoms in patients with RA and atlantoaxial instability. In that study, 60% of 32 patients had an AADI that did not equal or exceed the common operative criteria of 9 mm, despite these patients being paralyzed. In contrast, a PADI of less than or equal to 13 mm was present in all but one of these patients. The PADI was also predictive of neurological recovery in these patients; no patients with a PADI less than 10 mm showed any substantial return of neurological function. The study concluded that patients with a PADI of 14 mm or less should undergo operative stabilization [2, 4]. The odontoid or open-mouth view shows the C1–C2 articulation. The distance between the medial border of the lateral mass of C1 and the dens should be symmetrical. There should be less than 2 mm of lateral overhang of C1 on C2. A combined lateral overhang of greater than 6.9 mm is never normal and may represent a Jefferson fracture or rupture of the transverse ligament in a Jefferson fracture (Fig. 3.6). The C1–C2 articulations should be parallel, with preserved height and no narrowing or sclerosis. The border of the dens should be smooth and rounded, with no cortical disruption.

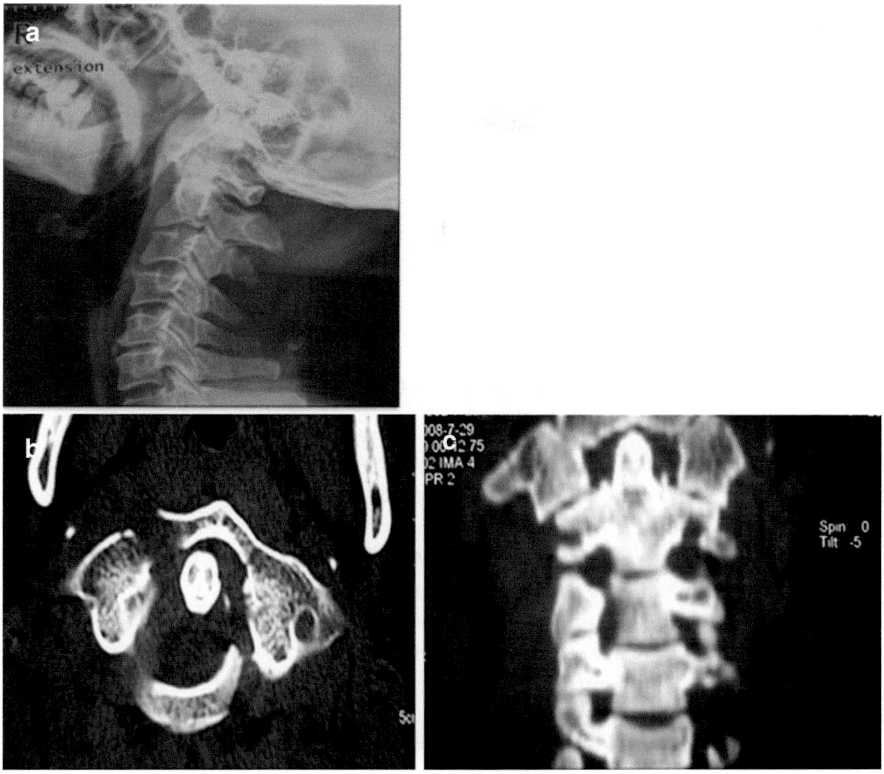

Fig. 3.7 A 25-year-old male patient reported neck pain after being involved in a traffic accident. (**a**) A lateral radiograph showing a subtle discontinuity of the dorsal arch of C1. This finding was not apparent on two other lateral radiographs. The absence of prevertebral soft tissue swelling at C1 does not exclude an acute fracture. (**b**) Bone algorithm technique axial CT at C1 showing several fractures of the anterior and posterior arches of C1. The atlantoaxial distance is not normal. (**c**) A 2D-CT coronal reconstruction image showing the right lateral mass of C1 with obvious displacement, providing a clearer image than the radiograph in (**a**)

3.3.2 Computed Tomography (CT)

CT remains the most sensitive imaging method to evaluate fractures of the upper cervical spine. In a prospective study of post-trauma patients, CT used as a primary screening tool had a sensitivity of 84% to detect upper cervical injury [5]. CT is also cost effective as a primary screening tool, especially in high- and moderate-risk patients [6]. With the added benefit of sagittal and coronal reconstructed images, CT has immense power to demonstrate complex fracture patterns not easily seen on standard radiography and on the axial images, especially at the occipitocervical junction (Fig. 3.7). In particular, the distance between the medial border of the lateral mass of C1 and the dens should be shown more clearly on the coronal reconstruction imaging than on plain radiography.

The availability of intraoperative CT scanning, such as the Medtronic O-arm and the Siemens Iso-C, combined with better image guidance software, allows real-time assessment of fracture displacement and reduction. This technology is especially useful in patients who are difficult to image because of their size or associated injuries. When combined with intraoperative image guidance software, internal fixation can be placed more precisely and safely than with traditional fluoroscopic imaging.

3.3.3 Magnetic Resonance Imaging (MRI)

MRI is not as good as CT or plain radiographs to identify and evaluate cervical fractures. Katzberg and colleagues [7] reported that for acute fractures, MRI had a weighted average sensitivity of 43%, compared with 48% for conventional radiography. Vaccaro and colleagues [8] also noted that MRI is not cost effective as a screening device in patients without a neurological deficit.

Despite its inadequacies in evaluating bony detail, MRI is unsurpassed for the assessment of soft tissue elements in the cervical spine. These structures include the intervertebral disc, ligamentous structures, and the spinal cord itself [9]. MRI is much more sensitive and specific than plain radiographs for the evaluation of a prevertebral hematoma. MRI is also useful to detect spinal cord hemorrhage, which, if present, carries a poor prognosis for neurological recovery. Acute hemorrhage has a low signal intensity on T2-weighted images (secondary to intracellular deoxyhemoglobin) and becomes hyperintense over the next several days after it becomes converted to extracellular methemoglobin. MRI diffusion studies allow a more accurate assessment of the degree of spinal stenosis. These diffusion studies assess the flow of cerebrospinal fluid (CSF) around the spinal cord at an area of constriction. If the degree of spinal stenosis is severe, CSF flow is significantly compromised [9].

3.4 Treatments

3.4.1 Nonsurgical Treatment

3.4.1.1 Pharmacotherapy

Pharmacotherapies target not the AAI itself but the underlying primary or associated disease, such as RA and Grisel's syndrome. In addition, NSAIDs can be used when the local pain is significant. Steroids may be considered in cases associated with severe neurological deficits; however, this remains controversial, and they are no longer recommended for routine use in spinal cord trauma [10]. Pharmacotherapies also include therapies to treat the complications of SCI, such as pulmonary infection and electrolyte disturbance.

3.4.1.2 Immobilization

Immobilization, including cervical collar, traction, and a Halo-vest, can be adapted to most traumatic AAIs. As routine initial treatments, a hard cervical collar is used for protection until a thorough neurological examination is completed and appropriate imaging is obtained. In patients with displacement, reduction should be obtained by traction or by a halo-vest. In fact, most traumatic AAIs respond well to a regular course of immobilization treatments for 6–12 weeks. Although long-term skull traction and the halo-vest are tolerated poorly by patients and are associated with morbidity, in most cases, these treatments save patients from the permanent loss of most upper cervical motion resulting from upper cervical fusion.

Cervical Collar

Cervical collars, such as the Necloc, the stiff neck collar, and the Philadelphia brace, offer the patient more safety especially during their out-of-bed activities. Most of the orthoses restrict flexion and extension better than lateral bending. However, they still allow significant motion of the cervical spine and have only limited effect on restricting motion of the cervical spine. A cervical collar is used routinely for first-line assistance, for pre-hospitalization, and for postoperative protection.

Skeletal Skull Traction

Skeletal skull traction plays an important role in stabilizing and realigning the cervical spine in the initial phase, and is indicated mainly in cases of facet subluxation or dislocation, and in burst-type fractures. But traction is not suitable for patients with distractive injuries or with certain skull fractures. Before operation for C1–C2 dislocation, skull traction should be routinely performed. Whether or not reduction of C1–C2 is achieved plays a decisive role in the surgical operation planning.

Halo-vest

The halo-vest was first described by Nickel and Perry [11] in 1959. It is a rigid ring that attaches to the outer cortex of the cranium through four sharp-tipped pins. It plays a key role in damage control management of cervical injuries. It can protect the injured neck, offer traction to the spine, maintain the reduction, and provide spinal stability until the trauma is healed. In certain cases, a halo-vest can avoid more progressive surgery, but it remains a controversial treatment because of its low fixation efficiency and high complication rate including pin loosening, penetration, migration, skull fracture, scalp infection, and cerebral hemorrhage [12]. Patients inevitably feel inconvenienced in their daily life for a long time.

3.4.2 Surgical Treatment

Surgical treatment of AAI comprises two main techniques: treatment of specific upper cervical diseases and/or trauma and C1–C2 fusion techniques. In general, osteosynthesis is always preferred over arthrodesis, which inevitably results in major loss of cervical motion. Only for patients with ligament damage that is thought incapable of healing should surgical internal fixation and fusion be considered. In cases where C1–C2 reduction is achieved preoperatively, atlantoaxial fusion is sufficient. Otherwise, irreducible C1–C2 dislocation (which should be confirmed under general anesthesia preoperatively) requires occipital-cervical fusion with excision of the C1 posterior arch.

3.4.2.1 Treatment of Upper Cervical Diseases and/or Trauma Leading to AAI

Odontoid Fracture

The Anderson and Alonzo classification [13] is widely accepted and predicts prognosis. Type I injuries are avulsion fractures of the lateral dens tip, secondary to the alar ligament. Therefore, they may be associated with occipitocervical instability. Type II injuries are fractures through the waist of the dens. The fracture occurs through cortical bone having a small cross-sectional area. Significant anterior or posterior displacement can occur. Type III injuries represent fractures that extend into the body of C-2. They have a broad fracture surface of the trabecular bone and, therefore, a good prognosis. Displacement, if present, is usually anterior.

Type I injuries, which are rare, should be evaluated carefully for occipitoatlantal instability. If present, they are treated by occipitocervical fusion. Stable type I injuries are treated by collar immobilization for 6 weeks.

The treatment of type II injuries is controversial. Nonoperative treatment is associated with a high failure rate, whereas operative care can lead to loss of range of motion or other iatrogenic complications. Type II fractures without immobilization have a near 100% chance of non-union. In addition, the halo-vest can only achieve a 15–85% union rate, which therefore requires internal fixation. For the transverse fractures without comminution and with less than 4–5 mm initial displacement, direct odontoid screw fixation can be performed. This has the advantage of being a direct fracture repair, thus maintaining atlantoaxial motion. When the fracture line runs parallel to the screw trajectory, a posterior C1–C2 fusion is indicated.

Type III fractures heal in 95% of cases when treated using the halo-vest. Other studies have demonstrated a small series of patients that healed successfully using a cervicothoracic brace. Unstable type III fractures or treatment failures are treated by a posterior C1–C2 fusion. Type III fractures are a relative contraindication for odontoid screw fixation.

Jefferson Fractures

Based on radiographic assessment of the integrity of the transverse ligament, bursting atlantal fractures were subdivided into stable and unstable types. Bursting fractures associated with an offset greater than 6.9 mm are considered as unstable.

Furthermore, according to the Dickman classification [2], nonoperative treatment should be used initially for type II injuries of the transverse ligament [14]. For type I and type II patients who have non-union with persistent instability after 3–5 months of immobilization, surgical treatment should be performed in the early stage. And radiographic follow-up of type II injuries is required to detect patients requiring delayed operative intervention.

However, considering the low fixation efficacy, the high complication rate, and the inconvenience of the halo-vest, increasing numbers of authors [15, 16] suggest direct posterior C1–C2 fusion for unstable Jefferson fractures.

Os Odontoideum

Os odontoideum often lead to AAI. Depending on its severity, patients may experience neck pain, limited neck mobility, or even neurological dysfunction such as sensory defects or gait abnormalities. Severe os odontoideum cases may cause spinal cord compression, leading to paralysis or even death. It is now widely accepted that os odontoideum with pain, C1–C2 dislocation, or neurological deficit should undergo a surgical intervention in the form of reduction and fusion because there is no effective and reliable nonoperative method to stabilize the atlantoaxial joint.

The treatment of asymptomatic os odontoideum remains controversial because the prognoses vary with different natural histories. Earlier authors [17, 18] believe that conventional treatment could be safe and effective. However, in patients with previously undiagnosed os odontoideum, there are reports of sudden death and significant neurological complications caused by minor trauma. Besides, even mild C1–C2 instability might thicken the periodontoid soft tissue mass because of chronic excessive stress. And hypertrophy of the periodontoid soft tissue mass may lead to spinal cord compression. Klimo et al. [19] insisted that all patients with os odontoideum should undergo surgical stabilization. They believed that the patients could be safe from potentially spinal cord injury only if C1–C2 fusion was achieved.

Rheumatoid Arthritis

RA is a chronic inflammatory disease of the synovial membrane associated with damage to the bone and cartilaginous and ligamentous structures. Involvement of the cervical spine is common. In the upper cervical spine, involvement of the ligamentous apparatus can result in severe complications including AAI and upward migration of the dens.

Most authors accept that clinical and radiological follow-up is enough for patients with radiographically confirmed instability, but with no or only mild neck pain, and no neurological symptoms. Surgical procedures with decompression, reduction, and stabilization are indicated if there is severe pain, progressive instability, or definite neurological symptoms. Atlantoaxial fusion in RA brings advantages including pain reduction and restoration of anatomical configuration, and thus subsequent complications, such as myelopathy caused by continuous compression of the spinal cord, can be avoided.

Precise timing of surgical intervention for C1–C2 instability from RA remains a matter of debate. Some authors suggest that surgical intervention is only indicated in case of atlantoaxial instability of more than 8 or 9 mm of the anterior ADI. However, the patients are always at risk of mortality because they cannot afford to sustain an accidental injury before surgery for reliable fixation. And too late interventions have proved to worsen the prognosis.

3.4.2.2 Techniques of Posterior C1–C2 Fusion

Wiring Techniques

Wiring techniques include Gallie (described by Grob [20]), Brooks and Jenkins [21], and Dickman [22] are the classical approaches to C1–C2 fusion. Until the screw techniques, which are much superior to wiring techniques appeared, wiring techniques are applied widely. They are fast, simple, and convenient. However, the use of wiring techniques requires an intact posterior lamina; the sublaminar passage of the wire risks spinal cord injury. The major disadvantage of wiring techniques is the poor mechanical stability, which contributes to its high rate of non-union, and the patients require longer periods of external postoperative immobilization [23]. Currently they are rarely used alone for atlantoaxial fixation.

Interlaminar Clamp Techniques

Interlaminar clamps used in atlantoaxial fixation were first reported in 1984 and were called the Halifax technique [24]. These techniques provide similar stability to that of the Brooks-Jenkins technique, but they avoid the disadvantage of sublaminar wires. Despite of excellent anteroposterior stability, clamp fixation provides poor rotational stability and allows translational deformation along the sagittal plane.

Thus, non-union and hardware failure comprise the majority of complications of the interlaminar clamps technique.

Atlantoaxial Transarticular Screw Technique

Atlantoaxial transarticular screw fixation for atlantoaxial stabilization was first reported by Jeanneret and Magerl in 1992 [25]. The screws are inserted through bilateral atlantoaxial lateral joints, and Gallie technique is usually performed to secure the bone graft. Atlantoaxial transarticular screw fixation provides excellent stability and achieves a high fusion rate. It is generally considered the "gold standard" of posterior atlantoaxial fusion.

Limitation of C1–C2 transarticular screw fixation is that it requires preliminary reduction of the atlantoaxial joint, and it is difficult to be instrumented in patients with thoracic kyphosis. Transarticular screw is also limited by anatomical variations of the foramen transversarium in up to 20% of patients. And the screw has potential risk of injury to the spinal cord, the vertebral artery, and the hypoglossal nerve.

C1–C2 Screw-Rod (Plate) System

The C1–C2 screw-plate system was first described by Goel and Laheri [26] in 1994. The system was comprised of bilateral C1 lateral mass screws and bilateral C2 pars screws; and the ipsilateral C1 and C2 screws are connected by a metal plate.

Harms and Melcher [27] later modified this technique into a screw-rod system which became more popularized. C1–C2 screw-rod (plate) system provides rigid immobilization and produces excellent clinical results. Compared with atlantoaxial transarticular screw technique, C1–C2 screw-rod (plate) system is not limited to preliminary reduction of the atlantoaxial joint, and it can provide intraoperative reduction by screw-rod manipulation.

References

1. Blacksin MF, Lee HJ. Frequency and significance of fractures of the upper cervical spine detected by CT in patients with severe neck trauma. AJR Am J Roentgenol. 1995;165(5):1201–4.
2. Dickman CA, Greene KA, Sonntag VK. Injuries involving the transverse atlantal ligament: classification and treatment guidelines based upon experience with 39 injuries. Neurosurgery. 1996;38(1):44–50.
3. Boden SD. Rheumatoid arthritis of the cervical spine. Surgical decision making based on predictors of paralysis and recovery. Spine (Phila PA 1976). 1994;19(20):2275–80.
4. Oda T, Panjabi MM, Crisco JJ 3rd. Three-dimensional translational movements of the upper cervical spine. J Spinal Disord. 1991;4(4):411–9.
5. Radcliff K, et al. CT and MRI-based diagnosis of craniocervical dislocations: the role of the occipitoatlantal ligament. Clin Orthop Relat Res. 2012;470(6):1602–13.

6. Monckeberg JE, et al. CT scan study of atlantoaxial rotatory mobility in asymptomatic adult subjects: a basis for better understanding C1-C2 rotatory fixation and subluxation. Spine (Phila PA 1976). 2009;34(12):1292–5.
7. Katzberg RW, et al. Acute cervical spine injuries: prospective MR imaging assessment at a level 1 trauma center. Radiology. 1999;213(1):203–12.
8. Kurd MF, et al. Magnetic resonance imaging following spine trauma. JBJS Rev. 2015;3:10.
9. Bae YJ, et al. Cervical compressive myelopathy: flow analysis of cerebrospinal fluid using phase-contrast magnetic resonance imaging. Eur Spine J. 2017;26(1):40–8.
10. Bydon M, et al. The current role of steroids in acute spinal cord injury. World Neurosurg. 2014;82(5):848–54.
11. Nickel VL, et al. The halo. A spinal skeletal traction fixation device. J Bone Joint Surg Am. 1968;50(7):1400–9.
12. Lind B, Sihlbom H, Nordwall A. Halo-vest treatment of unstable traumatic cervical spine injuries. Spine (Phila PA 1976). 1988;13(4):425–32.
13. Anderson LD, D'Alonzo RT. Fractures of the odontoid process of the axis. J Bone Joint Surg Am. 1974;56(8):1663–74.
14. Lee TT, Green BA, Petrin DR. Treatment of stable burst fracture of the atlas (Jefferson fracture) with rigid cervical collar. Spine (Phila PA 1976). 1998;23(18):1963–7.
15. Guo X, et al. Bilateral atlas laminar hook combined with transarticular screw fixation for an unstable bursting atlantal fracture. Arch Orthop Trauma Surg. 2009;129(9):1203–9.
16. Kamal Y, et al. Atlas and axis injuries role of Halovest. Int J Health Sci (Qassim). 2014;8(4):335–45.
17. Dai L, et al. Os odontoideum: etiology, diagnosis, and management. Surg Neurol. 2000;53(2):106–8. discussion 108–9.
18. Spierings EL, Braakman R. The management of os odontoideum. Analysis of 37 cases. J Bone Joint Surg (Br). 1982;64(4):422–8.
19. Klimo P Jr, et al. Os odontoideum: presentation, diagnosis, and treatment in a series of 78 patients. J Neurosurg Spine. 2008;9(4):332–42.
20. Grob D, et al. Biomechanical evaluation of four different posterior atlantoaxial fixation techniques. Spine (Phila PA 1976). 1992;17(5):480–90.
21. Brooks AL, Jenkins EB. Atlanto-axial arthrodesis by the wedge compression method. J Bone Joint Surg Am. 1978;60(3):279–84.
22. Dickman CA, et al. The interspinous method of posterior atlantoaxial arthrodesis. J Neurosurg. 1991;74(2):190–8.
23. Coyne TJ, et al. C1-C2 posterior cervical fusion: long-term evaluation of results and efficacy. Neurosurgery. 1995;37(4):688–92. discussion 692–3.
24. Holness RO, et al. Posterior stabilization with an interlaminar clamp in cervical injuries: technical note and review of the long term experience with the method. Neurosurgery. 1984;14(3):318–22.
25. Jeanneret B, Magerl F. Primary posterior fusion C1/2 in odontoid fractures: indications, technique, and results of transarticular screw fixation. J Spinal Disord. 1992;5(4):464–75.
26. Goel A, Laheri V. Plate and screw fixation for atlanto-axial subluxation. Acta Neurochir. 1994;129(1–2):47–53.
27. Harms J, Melcher RP. Posterior C1-C2 fusion with polyaxial screw and rod fixation. Spine (Phila PA 1976). 2001;26(22):2467–71.

Chapter 4
Basic Concept of Translational Medicine

Xiang Guo and Jun Liu

Abstract This section introduces the basic concepts of translational medicine. According to the research results of Tufts University, translation medicine can be divided into four phrases. Using these four phases, clinical problems identified by clinicians can be solved, and the results can be transferred and applied to produce new clinical treatment devices or methods. As an academic research method, translational medicine promotes and speeds up the translation from basic research to clinical application.

"What is translational medicine?." Some researchers define translational medicine as from the lab to the disease (bench-to-bedside) and the development of new drugs, instruments, and treatment methods for patients. Other researchers consider that translational research is applied to practices, including prevention and health administration.

Breaking away from single studies or limited cooperation modes and advocating making patients the central focus, translational medicine emphasizes multidisciplinary cooperation and full realization of research potential. The core of translational medicine is to translate medical biological research results quickly and effectively into theories, techniques, methods, and drugs can be applied in clinical practice. In addition, translational medicine bridges the gap between the laboratory and the ward to realize two-way conversion of basic and clinical research.

According to research results of Tufts University, translation medicine was divided into four phrases [1]:

X. Guo (✉)
Department of Orthopedics, Changzheng Hospital, Shanghai, China

J. Liu
Department of Orthopedics, The Second Affiliated Hospital, Nanjing Medical University, Jiangsu, China

B. Ni et al. (eds.), *Atlantoaxial Fixation Techniques*, Translational Medicine Research, https://doi.org/10.1007/978-981-10-7889-7_4

4.1 Translation Phase 1 (T1)

To apply basic research results in a limited number of patients, usually in the form of case studies and phase I or II clinical trials. In addition, T1 validates whether a newly developed therapy can be used for a small number of patients in a hospital.

4.2 Translation Phrase 2 (T2)

To apply basic research results into a larger number of patients, usually in the form of phase III and IV clinical trials, and some observational and investigative studies. Phase 2 validates whether a new therapy developed in the laboratory can be used in a large number of patients in several hospitals, involving a few hundred even thousands of patients.

4.3 Translation Phrase 3 (T3)

Positive results from T2 can be carried forward into T3. This phase determines whether a newly developed therapy can be used for larger number of patients by spreading a series of studies and trials among different hospitals and laboratories, at the same time focusing on clinical problems and phase obstacles related to the new therapy.

4.4 Translation Phrase 4 (T4)

If the results of T1–T3 are valid, T4 can be conducted. This phase involves a series of policy researches, aimed at finding the best way to promote and apply the new therapy among clinicians and patients.

Traditionally, hospitals and doctors passively receive medical devices from manufacturers. The manufacturers develop new devices and provide them to hospitals via distributors, and the doctors use the products to cure patients. However, this is only part of the development process. Original ideas for new devices often result from clinical practices of doctors, who obtain such inspiration while treating patients, leading to improvements or innovations of existing therapies. Usually, these thoughts and ideas need to be realized in the form of new devices, which when developed, lead to improvements to existing therapies. This generates a corresponding market demand for such improvements. Companies can increase demand by gathering market data, inputting resources, cooperating with doctors to develop products, and using suitable distributors to maximize market penetration. As the new products are used by doctors, other innovations are conceived, creating a beneficial cycle for the entire industry.

In the modern information-based society, the development, production, evaluation, and distribution of products have experienced significant changes. For medical devices, massive data mining and accumulation have provided a solid basis for treatment; the development of industrial design and 3D printing techniques has shortened the research cycle significantly; and FEM and biomechanical experiments have assured the reliability of new products. These technological innovations have shortened the development time of medical devices. However, the economical and intelligence resources requirements are even more important. Hence, combining a devices' advantages and the integration of superior resources becomes one of the most important methods to develop medical devices.

For orthopedic devices, the cooperation of the doctor and device manufacturer is particularly important. With orthopedic devices, doctors have the most knowledge to determine the requirements of the products. In cooperation with engineers, doctors can transfer their thoughts into practical designs and, eventually, products. This has become a routine method in the orthopedics industry in recent years.

Unfortunately, not all ideas can become products. Product development is usually based on a company's strategy. Figure 4.1 shows the three main concerns of a company: market requirements, technique feasibility, and company benefits. The product can only be developed when all three concerns are satisfied. Market requirements include factors such as clinical demand, therapy innovation, or product regeneration. Technique feasibility includes support from existing materials, techniques, laws and regulations, therapeutic recognition, doctors' operative skills, and company resources. The company benefits usually mean long-term profitability after resource input. The physical development is performed using research and

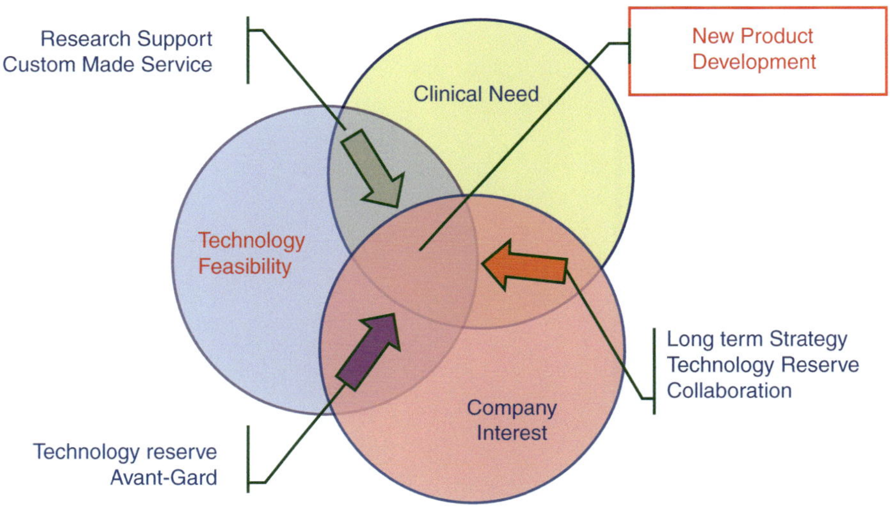

Fig. 4.1 Potential R&D projects

development programs. R&D programs comprise two parts: research programs and product development programs. Even when the main concerns are not all satisfied, the company will support research programs to enhance collaboration with doctors, to explore new technical availability, or to increase the R&D ability of the company.

Therefore, for a leading hospital, it is important to find a high-quality device manufacturer to integrate resource advantages and to provide strong R&D support to develop new devices. Thus, hospitals can provide better services to patients by getting timely feedback, turning thoughts into products faster, and making products more reliable. The company can then benefit socially and economically by gathering therapeutic experiences, increasing R&D efficiency, and shortening the development time cycles.

Translational medicine can improve the translation from basic research to clinical application effectively and rapidly via the cooperation of the doctor and device manufacturer. By contrast, considering the clinical problem to be the main direction of basic research can integrate basic research with related applicable fields systematically and scientifically, such as clinical medicine, nursing, and prevention. Furthermore, translational medicine accelerates the development of applied science and produces fundamental changes in the development medicine in the new century. The patients are the biggest beneficiaries of the translation of the results of basic research into clinical treatment.

Reference

1. Zerhouni EA. Translational and clinical science – time for a new vision. New Engl J Med. 2005;353:1621–3.

Part II

Established Posterior Atlantoaxial Fixation Techniques

Abstract

This section describes the traditional atlantoaxial fusion techniques and their integrated innovation. The first chapter mainly reviews the traditional posterior atlanto-axial fusion techniques including sublaminar wiring/cable technique, interlaminar clamps technique, transarticular screw fixation technique, and Cl–C2 segmental fixation techniques. Meanwhile, the biomechanics of different techniques and their advantages and disadvantages are analyzed. In the following three chapters, an integration modification of traditional posterior atlantoaxial fixation technique—"Hook Screw" fixation technique is presented, including its design, biomechanics, clinical outcomes, and limitations. The fifth chapter focuses on the basic principle of the translational medicine and presents the translation of posterior "hook-nail" atlanto-axial fixation. In the last chapter, some atlantoaxial personalized fixation techniques are described to conquer atlantoaxial anatomy variant.

Chapter 5
Advantages and Disadvantages of Traditional Atlantoaxial Fusion Techniques

Xuhua Lu and Tianming Xu

Abstract For C1–C2 instability, the primary goal of treatment is to reconstruct the normal C1–C2 alignment and achieve solid bone fusion, avoiding deterioration of the neurological function. Conservative management is associated with significant segmental movement at C1–C2 but results in relatively low fusion rates when used alone. Therefore, surgical treatment with internal fixation is generally used to promote higher fusion rates. Anterior and posterior techniques for stabilization of the C1–C2 segments have been developed during the last several decades. C1–C2 fixations from the posterior approach are the mainstays of surgical treatment for atlantoaxial instability. This chapter describes the traditional posterior atlantoaxial fusion techniques and their advantages and disadvantages.

5.1 Posterior Atlantoaxial Fusion Techniques

5.1.1 Sublaminar Wiring/Cable Techniques

The first successful treatment of C1–C2 instability was achieved by Mixter and Osgood [1] in 1910. In this procedure, C1 posterior arch was fixed to C2 spinous process by using a silk thread. In 1939, Gallie [2] was the first to describe such a technique. Since then, several sublaminar wire/cable techniques have been described. Among of these techniques, three basic sublaminar wire or cable fixation techniques, the Brooks [3], Gallie [2], and Sonntag techniques [4], are commonly used for C1–C2 fixation (Fig. 5.1).

X. Lu (✉)
Department of Orthopedics, Changzheng Hospital, Shanghai, China
e-mail: xuhualu@hotmail.com

T. Xu
Department of Orthopedics, No. 455 Hospital of PLA, Shanghai, China

B. Ni et al. (eds.), *Atlantoaxial Fixation Techniques*, Translational Medicine Research, https://doi.org/10.1007/978-981-10-7889-7_5

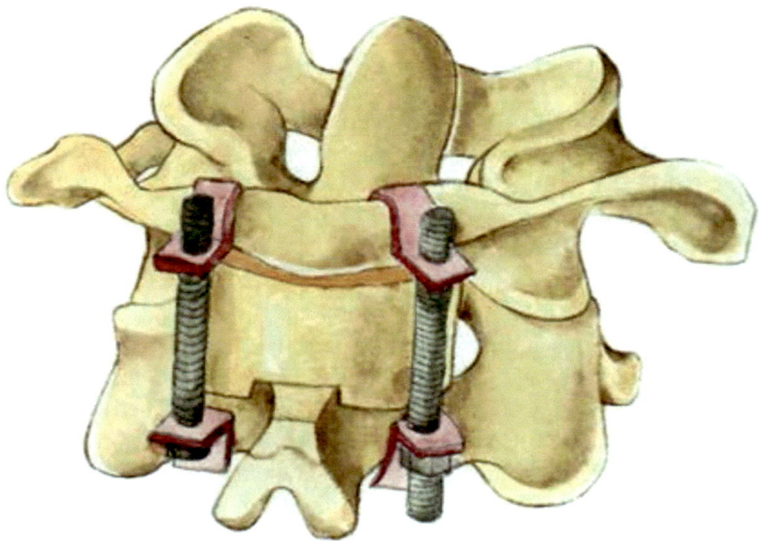

Fig. 5.1 Posterior sublaminar the interlaminar clamp technique

5.1.1.1 The Gallie Technique

This C1–C2 arthrodesis technique, first described by Gallie [2] in 1939, involves the placement of a wire under C1 that attached to C2 spinous process below using an intervening bone graft. The graft is typically a corticocancellous iliac crest bone which is notched caudally to contour the spinous process of C2 during compression.

5.1.1.2 The Brooks and Jenkins Technique

In 1978, Brooks and Jenkins [3] presented a modified wire fusion technique, with bone grafts being placed between C1 posterior arch and C2 lamina on both sides. Bilateral sublaminar wires are passed under C1 posterior arch and C2 lamina to secure the bone grafts bilaterally. In their technique, a single wire was used on each side, while two sublaminar wires were used in the following technique modified by Griswold et al. [5].

5.1.1.3 The Sonntag Technique

Dickman et al. [4] described the Sonntag technique in 1991.The inferior edge of C1 lamina and the superior edge of C2 spinous process and lamina are firstly decorticated. Then a bicortical bone graft is wedged between C1 lamina and C2 spinous process and lamina. The bone graft is secured by passing wires under C1 lamina and around the base of C2 spinous process.

5.1.2 The Interlaminar Clamp Technique

In 1975, Tucker [6] described the Halifax clamp technique. The Halifax clamp system comprises two fitted J-shaped interlaminar clamps with an intervening tightening screw. The threaded upper clamp is placed over the superior edge of C1 dorsal ring, and an unthreaded caudal clamp is placed under the inferior edge of C2 lamina. The clamps are then sequentially tightened while ensuring proper engagement of the hooks with the C1–C2 dorsal elements. An interspinous graft is secured between C1 dorsal arch and C2 lamina and spinous process under the compression provided by the clamps.

5.1.3 Transarticular Screw Fixation

Magerl [7] firstly described C1–C2 transarticular screw fixation technique. The entry point on C2 is 2 mm lateral from the medial edge of the facet and 3 mm superior to the caudal edge. The screw is inserted across C1 and C2 articular surfaces and finally into C1 lateral mass (Fig. 5.2a, b). Sometimes, a percutaneous route is necessary to provide the proper trajectory, with a small stab incision at the thoracic area. Before operation, computed tomography (CT) scans and sagittal CT reconstruction should be used to confirm that there are no contraindications for the placement of C1–C2 transarticular screws. Bone or vascular deformity should be identified to avoid vertebral artery (VA) injury. It was reported that VA deformity existed in up to 20% of patients, precluding bilateral transarticular screw insertion [8]. If VA injury is encountered, a much safer fixation technique should be used on the opposite side. Gallie or Sonntag fusion technique also is often performed after the placement of screws to achieve solid bone fusion.

5.1.4 C1–C2 Segmental Fixation

5.1.4.1 C1 Lateral Mass Screw and C2 Pedicle/Pars Screw Fixation

Goel and Laheri [9] introduced a C1–C2 fixation technique using C1 lateral mass screws and C2 pedicle screws with plate fixation in 1994. Harms and Melcher [10] modified this technique by the placement of polyaxial-head screws inserted into the C1 lateral mass and the C2 pedicle/pars with bilateral rod fixation in 2001. The entry point for the C1 screw is at the middle of the junction of the C1 posterior arch and the midpoint of the posterior inferior part of the C1 lateral mass. The screw trajectory is slightly convergent and parallel to the posterior arch plane of C1, heading to C1 anterior arch (Fig. 5.3). An alternative starting point to that described by Harms and Melcher [10] is located on the posterolateral arch of C1, overlying the lateral mass. The screw is inserted into the pedicle analog, rather than beneath it. This starting point eliminates the need to retract the C2 nerve root and does not require the same extent of inferior dissection through the C1–C2 venous plexus.

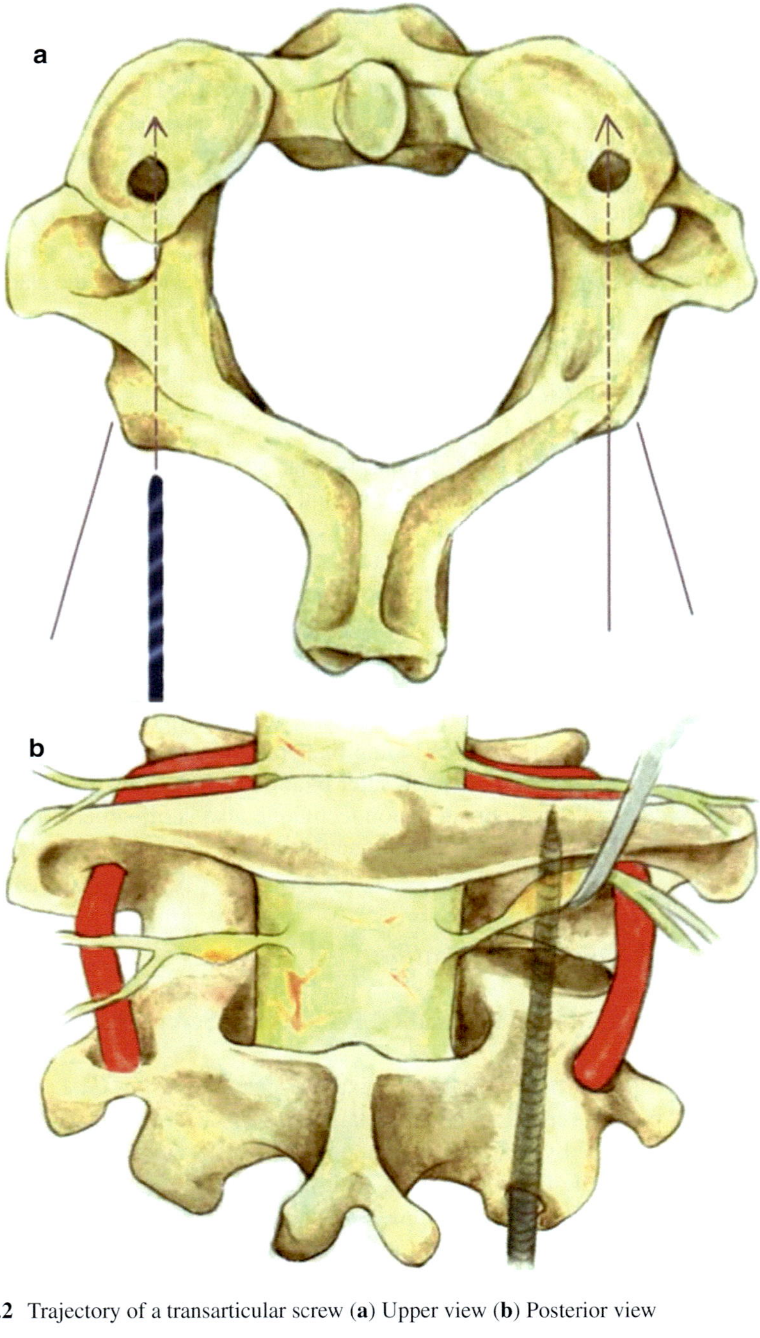

Fig. 5.2 Trajectory of a transarticular screw (**a**) Upper view (**b**) Posterior view

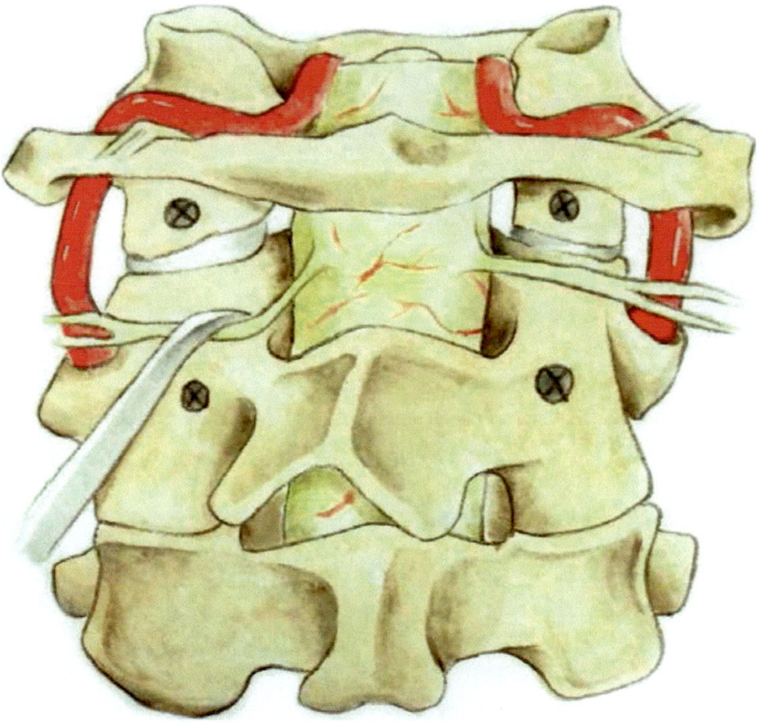

Fig. 5.3 Entry points of the C1 lateral mass screw and the C2 pedicle screw

This technique brings the screw closer to the overlying VA; therefore, proximal dissection to identify the top of the ring and protection of the VA are advised before cannulation and screw placement. The entry point for the C2 pedicle screw is in the inferior part of the C2 lateral mass at the midpoint of the C2–C3 facet joint. The C2 pedicle screw is inserted in a cephalad and convergent direction guided by the medial and superior surface of C2 isthmus, respecting individual anatomical variations. C2 pars screw is inserted according to the method to implant transarticular screw; however, the screw is significantly shorter and does not reach the C1–C2 facet joint. The C2 pars screw may be used primarily or as an alternative when other C2 fixation options are not possible. For the bone graft, morselized autologous bone grafts can be inserted into the decorticated C1–C2 facet complexes or on the surface of decorticated C1 posterior arch and C2 laminar. For cases with odontoid fractures, the implants can be removed after bone fusion to retain C1–C2 rotation.

5.1.4.2 C1 Lateral Mass Screw and Crossed C2 Intralaminar Screw Fixation

In 2004, Wright [11] first described the C2 intralaminar screw technique. He inserted two polyaxial-head screws into C2 lamina bilaterally in a crossing way. The screw entry point is at the junction of lamina and the spinous process. If bilateral

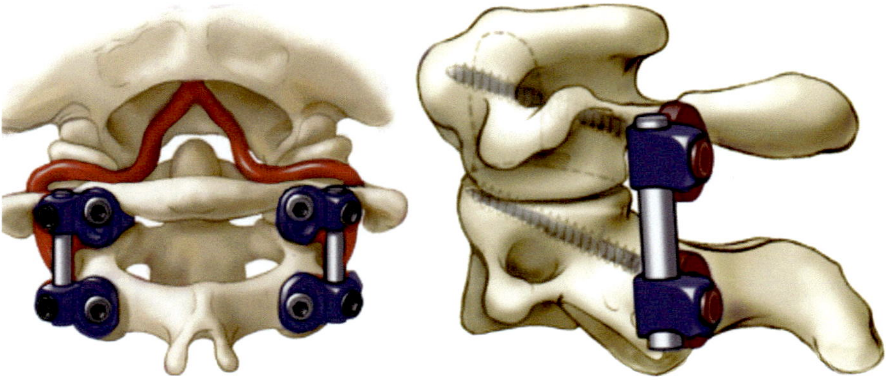

Fig. 5.4 Lateral and dorsal views of the C1 lateral mass screw and the C2 pedicle screw

Fig. 5.5 Intralaminar screws

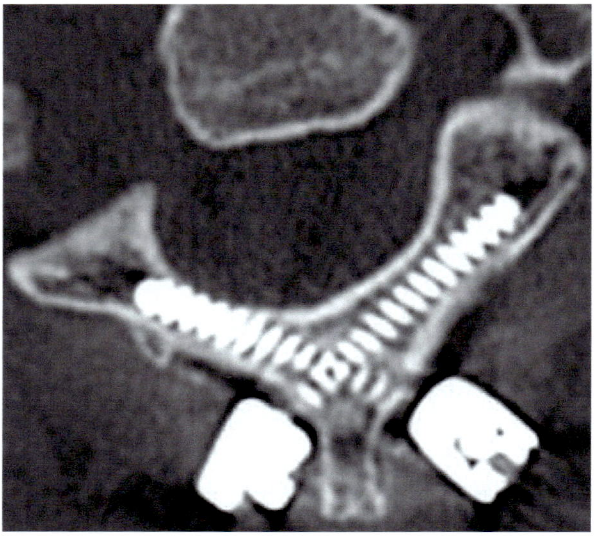

intralaminar C2 screw is to be used, the first screw should be inserted cranially while the second screw caudally to avoid screw trajectories intersection. The screw is directed within the contralateral lamina, not exceeding the dorsal or ventral cortex (intralaminar) (Fig. 5.4). The endpoint of C2 intralaminar screw is located just caudal to the junction between the lamina and the pars interarticularis. Ipsilateral screw heads of C1 and C2 are connected. For bone fusion, a tricortical autologous iliac crest bone graft can be harvested and inserted between decorticated C2 spinous process and C1 posterior arch. The morselized bone graft can also be used according to the abovementioned method in *C1 lateral mass screw and C2 pedicle/pars screw fixation* technique (Fig. 5.5).

5.2 Biomechanical Evaluation of Posterior C1–C2 Fixation Techniques

Long-term stability of the C1–C2 complex depends on bone fusion, which requires rigid limitation of C1–C2 motion. Therefore, biomechanics of different posterior C1–C2 techniques were evaluated by many studies.

In the study by Dickman et al. [12], the biomechanics of four different methods of C1–C2 cable fixation including the interspinous technique, the Brooks technique, and two variants of the Gallie technique were evaluated. After cyclic loading, all of the four techniques loosened. C1–C2 rotation and translation were significantly increased. However, they found that it was significantly better for the Brooks and interspinous methods to control C1–C2 motion than both Gallie techniques. There were no significant differences in C1–C2 motions between one of the Gallie techniques and unfixed destabilized specimens. During cyclic loading, the bone grafts shifted, reducing the effectiveness of the fixation technique. Therefore, they concluded that some adjunctive fixation should be used to strengthen the ability to control C1–C2 motion after C1–C2 cable fixation.

Naderi et al. [13] evaluated the biomechanics of four combinations of cables, grafts, and screw fixation at C1–C2. Posterior cable-graft constructs alone were less effective in controlling axial rotation and lateral bending compared with transarticular screws fixation. However, cable-graft constructs are more effective in control flexion and extension than stand-alone screw fixation techniques. Therefore, the authors concluded that an increased number of fixation points were associated with a significant decrease in the range of axial rotation and translation, confirming the biomechanical advantage of using as many C1–C2 fixation points as possible.

Melcher et al. [14] compared the acute stability produced by posterior C1–C2 segmental screw fixation with transarticular screw combined with wire techniques. They found that both screw techniques could significantly decrease motion in axial rotation and lateral bending compared with wiring techniques. There was no statistically significant difference between the two screw techniques in the control of C1–C2 motion.

Richter et al. [15] evaluated the biomechanics of six kinds of C1–C2 fixation techniques, including Gallie fixation, transarticular screw fixation, transarticular screw combined with Gallie fixation, transarticular screw with C1 claw, C2 isthmic screw with C1 claw, and C1 lateral mass screw with C2 isthmic screw. They found that the transarticular screws provided the best restriction of axial rotation and lateral bending. Transarticular screws combined with Gallie or C1 claws, a three-point fixation, additionally restricted the motion in flexion-extension, with the most rigid fixation afforded by transarticular screws combined with C1 claws. The other techniques, including C2 isthmic screws with C1 claws and C1 lateral mass screws with C2 isthmic screws, were less effective in the control of C1–C2 motions than the three-point fixations but were more effective than the Gallie fixation.

Gorek et al. [16] compared the acute atlantoaxial stability provided by intralaminar screws in C2 with that afforded by C2 pedicle screws. They found that there were no differences in acute atlantoaxial stability afforded by polyaxial screw-rod constructs that used C1 lateral mass screws combined with C2 pedicle/intralaminar screws.

Sim et al. [17] evaluated the biomechanics of five different posterior reconstructions that were usually used in the treatment of atlantoaxial instability. The fixation techniques included C1 lateral mass combined with C2 short/long pedicle screw or C2 intralaminar screw fixations, Sonntag's modified Gallie fixation, and C1–C2 transarticular screw combined with Sonntag's modified Gallie fixations. They found that C1–C2 transarticular screw combined with modified Gallie fixation, a three-point fixation technique, provided the highest stability in all directions of C1–C2 motion. The C1 lateral mass combined with C2 intralaminar screw fixation was less effective in the control of lateral bending. The Sonntag's modified Gallie fixation was less effective than the other fixation techniques in the control of C1–C2 lateral bending and rotation. There was no difference in obtaining immediate C1–C2 stability between C2 short pedicle screw and long pedicle screw fixation.

5.3 Advantages and Disadvantages of Traditional Posterior Atlantoaxial Fusion Techniques

5.3.1 Sublaminar Wiring/Cable Techniques

Posterior wiring/cable techniques share the advantages of surgeon familiarity, as well as fusion rates reported in the range of 60–100%. The main disadvantages of the procedures are the risk of neurological injury caused by wiring/cable placement and the lack of biomechanical stability attainable with this technique alone. To improve C1–C2 stability and bony fusion rates, an additional external or internal fixation is often needed. Furthermore, wiring/cable techniques can only be performed in cases with an intact C1 posterior arch and C2 lamina. They are not accessible for patients with posterior element fractures or that requiring posterior decompression. In addition, the C1–C2 complex should be reduced well before the use of sublaminar wires or cables to avoid spinal cord injury.

5.3.2 Interlaminar Clamp Technique

Interlaminar clamps do not require sublaminar passage and avoid the risk of neurological injury associated with wiring/cable techniques. Bone grafts can be inserted between C1 posterior arch and C2 lamina and secured directly by tightening the C1 and C2 clamps, and interlaminar clamps are relatively easy to apply. However, there are some disadvantages, including graft dislodgment into the spinal canal resulting in subsequent neural injury, construct failure caused by screw loosening, disengagement of laminar hooks, C1 dorsal arch fracture, and neurological injury secondary to canal stenosis as a result of the placement of the sublaminar hooks. In addition, the use of interlaminar clamps requires an intact lamina. For patients with posterior element fracture or patients needing laminectomy, clamp fixation cannot be performed. In biomechanics aspect, the construct has a low ability to resist counter anterior-posterior translation and rotational forces.

5.3.3 Transarticular Screw Fixation

Fixation of the C1–C2 complex with transarticular screws can provide immediate stabilization. It is not necessary for this technique to have a complete C1 posterior arch. In cases with an intact C1 posterior arch, a combination of bilateral transarticular screw fixation and bone graft with the Gallie technique, the three-point fixation, can provide not only the best restriction of rotation and lateral bending but also superior limitation of flexion and extension. However, there are some disadvantages to this technique, including the risk of VA injury, spinal cord injury, and hypoglossal nerve injury. In addition, it needs a steep learning curve and cannot be used in cases with non-reducible C1–C2 subluxations.

VA injury is one of the most serious complications with C1–C2 transarticular screw placement. In a study by Wright and Lauryssen [18], the rates of confirmed and suspected VA injuries were 2.4% and 1.7%, respectively. Neurological deficits due to VA injury happened in 3.7% of the patients with confirmed or suspected VA injuries. One patient (1.9%) died of a bilateral VA injury. Other complications included screw breakout/fracture, fusion failure, infection, and so on. Cadaveric studies revealed that transarticular screw could not be safely inserted in as many as 20% of patients due to an aberrant VA that indents or grooves the C2 pars interarticularis. Therefore, a CT scan and reconstruction should be done to identify the aberrant VA and to help determine the optimal screw trajectory to avoid the VA.

5.3.4 C1 Lateral Mass Screw and C2 Pars/Pedicle Screw Fixation

This technique is equivalent biomechanically to transarticular screw placement but with higher fusion rates. The advantage of this technique, compared with the transarticular screw technique or wiring techniques, is that anatomical C1–C2 alignment is not necessary before instrumentation. C1 and C2 screws can be inserted independently, and open reduction can be performed with the screw-rod system. The disadvantage of this technique also includes VA injury, although the risk is less than that in transarticular screw placement.

5.3.5 C2 Translaminar Screws

The placement of C2 translaminar screws is safe and relatively easy to perform. It avoids arterial injury, being safely inserted with no need of surgical navigation techniques at C2. However, the C1 lateral mass combined with C2 intralaminar screw fixation is less stable biomechanically than the C1 lateral mass screw with C2 pedicle/pars screw fixation and C1–C2 transarticular screw with posterior wiring fixation. Therefore, it is often used as an alternative treatment to C2 pars or pedicle screws. Additionally, it has the risk of neural injury if the lamina breached.

References

1. Mixter SJ, Osgood RB IV. Traumatic lesions of the atlas and axis. Ann Surg. 1910;51:193–207.
2. Gallie W. Fractures and dislocations of the cervical spine. Am J Surg. 1939;46:495–9.
3. Brooks AL, Jenkins EB. Atlanto-axial arthrodesis by the wedge compression method. J Bone Joint Surg Am. 1978;60:279–84.
4. Dickman CA, Sonntag VK, Papadopoulos SM, et al. The interspinous method of posterior atlantoaxial arthrodesis. J Neurosurg. 1991;74:190–8.
5. Griswold DM, Albright JA, Schiffman E, et al. Atlanto-axial fusion for instability. J Bone Joint Surg Am. 1978;60:285–92.
6. Tucker HH. Technical report: method of fixation of subluxed or dislocated cervical spine below C1–C2. Can J Neurol Sci. 1975;2:381–2.
7. Magerl F, Seeman PS. Stable posterior fusion of the atlas by transarticular screw fixation. In: Kehr P, Weidner A, editors. Cervical spine I. New York: Springer; 1987.
8. Paramore CG, Dickman CA, Sonntag VK. The anatomical suitability of the C1–2 complex for transarticular screw fixation. J Neurosurg. 1996;85:221–4.
9. Goel A, Laheri V. Plate and screw fixation for atlanto-axial subluxation. Acta Neurochir. 1994;129:47–53.
10. Harms J, Melcher RP. Posterior C1–C2 fusion with polyaxial screw and rod fixation. Spine. 2001;26:2467–71.
11. Wright NM. Posterior C2 fixation using bilateral, crossing C2 laminar screws: case series and technical note. J Spinal Disord Tech. 2004;17:158–62.
12. Dickman CA, Crawford NR, Paramore CG. Biomechanical characteristics of C1–2 cable fixations. J Neurosurg. 1996;85:316–22.
13. Naderi S, Crawford NR, Song GS, et al. Biomechanical comparison of C1–C2 posterior fixations. Cable, graft, and screw combinations. Spine. 1998;23:1946–55.
14. Melcher RP, Puttlitz CM, Kleinstueck FS, et al. Biomechanical testing of posterior atlantoaxial fixation techniques. Spine. 2002;27:2435–40.
15. Richter M, Schmidt R, Claes L, et al. Posterior atlantoaxial fixation: biomechanical in vitro comparison of six different techniques. Spine. 2002;27:1724–32.
16. Gorek J, Acaroglu E, Berven S, et al. Constructs incorporating intralaminar C2 screws provide rigid stability for atlantoaxial fixation. Spine. 2005;30:1513–8.
17. Sim HB, Lee JW, Park JT, et al. Biomechanical evaluations of various C1–C2 posterior fixation techniques. Spine. 2011;36:E401–7.
18. Wright NM, Lauryssen C. Vertebral artery injury in C1–2 transarticular screw fixation: results of a survey of the AANS/CNS section on disorders of the spine and peripheral nerves. American Association of Neurological Surgeons/Congress of Neurological Surgeons. J Neurosurg. 1998;88:634–40.

Chapter 6
Integration and Modification of the Traditional Posterior Atlantoaxial Fixation Technique: The "Hook+Screw" Fixation Technique

Mingfei Wang and Qi Liu

Abstract Posterior atlantoaxial fixation methods include many techniques from cable to screw-rod fixations. Established fixation techniques, including Gallie or Brooks, Apofix laminar clamp, Magerl screw, and atlas lateral mass screws combined with axial pedicle screw fixation, have their respective deficiencies, such as lower bone graft fusion rate and poorer biomechanical stability. To improve the biomechanical characteristics and clinical outcome of established techniques, we integrated the advantages of established techniques and developed a modified posterior atlantoaxial fixation technique, "Hook+Screw." This chapter focuses on the biomechanical evaluation and clinical outcome of this modified posterior atlantoaxial technique.

The atlantoaxial instability is an unusual disease which often results from trauma, rheumatoid arthritis, and congenital deformity in the craniocervical region [1]. Significant atlantoaxial instability is usually accompanied by dynamic life-threatening spinal cord compression. Conservative treatment methods composed by brace or cast vest often are inefficient for these patients because of recurrent atlantoaxial instability and appearance of dynamic spinal cord compression; therefore surgery intervention is considered a preferred treatment, from which patients can immediately achieve atlantoaxial stability and decompress spinal cord compression [1, 2].

M. Wang (✉)
Department of Orthopedics, Putuo Hospital, Shanghai University of Traditional Chinese Medicine, Shanghai, China
e-mail: wmf88@126.com

Q. Liu
Department of Orthopedics, The First Affiliated Hospital of Xiamen University, Xiamen, China

B. Ni et al. (eds.), *Atlantoaxial Fixation Techniques*, Translational Medicine Research, https://doi.org/10.1007/978-981-10-7889-7_6

From a biomechanical viewpoint, posterior fixation techniques of the atlantoaxial articulation are mainly divided into three types: one-point fixation, two-point fixation, and three-point fixation. One-point fixation merely restricts the motion of the spinal posterior structure (e.g., Gallie wiring and Halifax clamps). Two-point fixation restricts the motion of C1–C2 articulation with laterally placing C1–C2 transarticular screws. Three-point fixation includes the combination of the above two types, such as C1–C2 transarticular screw combined with Gallie fixation; thus this three-point fixation can stabilize the C1–C2 joint from both laterally and posteriorly. Some biomechanical studies have demonstrated that three-point fixation is superior to any other fixation methods [3, 4].

In 1986, Magerl et al. first introduced the C1–C2 transarticular screw fixation technique [5]. From that time, this technique is always considered to be the optimal choice for patients who need atlantoaxial fixation because of its excellent biomechanical and clinical results [5]. However, this technique still cannot provide efficient restriction to the three-dimensional motion of the atlantoaxial articulation because it is merely a two-point fixation. In order to further improve the biomechanical stability of fixation technique, the authors innovated a novel posterior atlantoaxial fixation technique "Hook+Screw" after researching deficits and advantages of established posterior atlantoaxial fixation techniques [6]. "Hook+Screw" technique integrated C1–C2 transarticular screws and C1 laminar hooks into a whole fixation system (Fig. 6.1), which can join to each other with a rod and transverse connectors to form a solid three-point fixation [6].

6.1 Biomechanical Testing of the "Hook+Screw" Atlantoaxial Fixation Technique

Although modification of this internal fixation theoretically can bring more solid fixation, the in vitro biomechanical test, as a golden test method, should be performed in fresh neck specimen to validate the stability of the modified atlantoaxial fixation via compared to usual atlantoaxial fixations. The detailed test procedure referred the paper of Xiang Guo [7].

The test results presented that the three-point fixation from TA+hook group has the minimal ROM value; moreover the C1 + C2 fixation has a higher ROM value compared with those three-point fixation techniques, but it is considered to be an alternative fixation technique for TA fixation technique. The biomechanical test result is considered as a precondition for clinical test of the modified fixation. By now, authors have already used the TA+hook internal fixation technique successfully to treat 87 patients. Results at 5-year follow-up showed optimal clinical outcomes. This demonstrated clearly that the TA+hook has a promising future as a modified fixation technique.

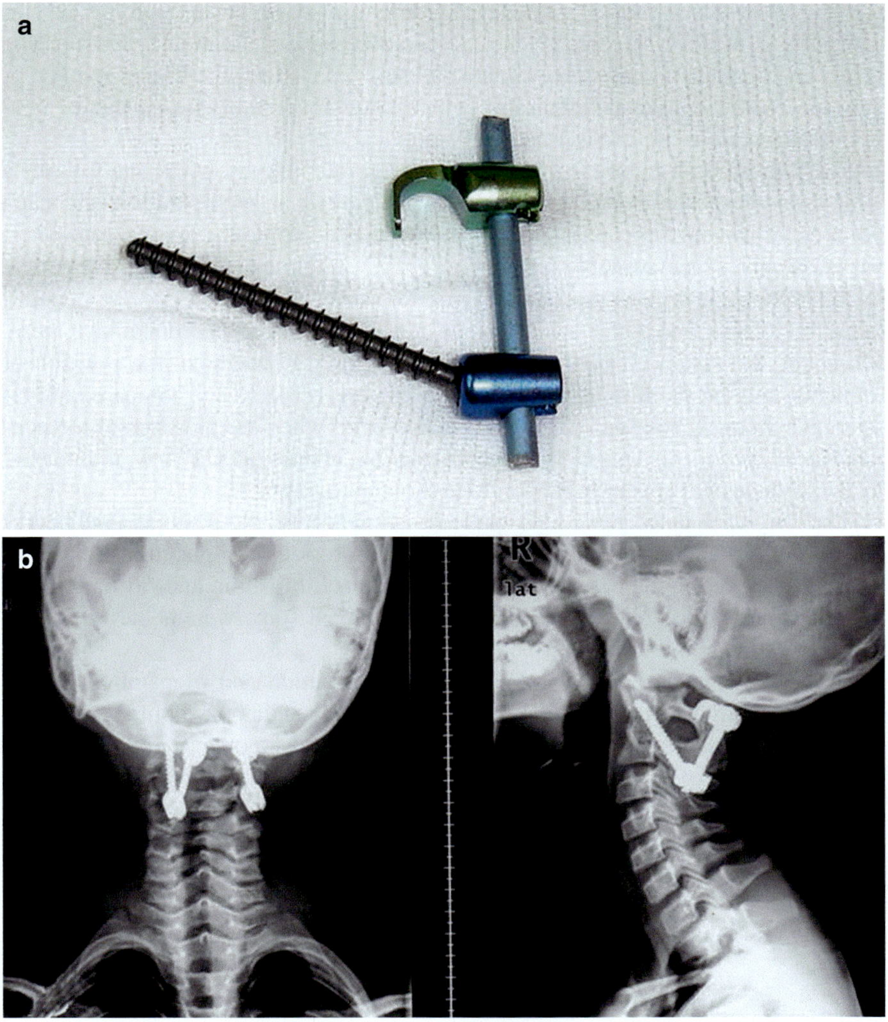

Fig. 6.1 The modified implant and postoperative radiographs of patient 1. A color photograph (**a**) shows the C1–C2 transarticular Hook+Screw implant. Postoperative lateral and anteroposterior view radiographs (**b**) demonstrate the satisfactory position of implants, as examined by the spinal surgery team during their outpatient follow-up

6.2 Clinical Outcome of the "Hook+Screw" Atlantoaxial Fixation Technique

From May 2006 to March 2010, this modified "Hook+Screw" technique has been used to treat 65 patients with reducible atlantoaxial dislocations. Recently, a retrospective clinical research [6] has been conducted to evaluate the clinical and radiological outcomes of this new fixation technique.

Clinical evaluation index, including symptom improvements, neurological status, and VAS scales, was recorded at pre-operation and each point of follow-up. The visual analog scale was used to evaluate patients' pain extent; the Ranawat myelopathy score and the myelopathy disability index were applied to assess patients' neurological function [6]. And any surgical complications were investigated.

The radiological materials, including cervical radiographs, MRI, and CT scans with three-dimensional reconstructions, were gained at pre-operation and each point of follow-up. Subsequently the specific data including the atlanto-dens interval (ADI), the space available for the cord (SAC), and the C1–C2 angle (the angle included by a line drawn parallel to the inferior aspect of C1 and a line drawn parallel to the inferior end plate of C2) were tested and compared to preoperative these. Moreover, the signal change of the spinal cord on T2 weighted, the position of implants, and the stability of atlantoaxial joint were, respectively, compared to preoperative those. A bone fusion was considered well when the presence of trabeculated bone occurs in the sagittal reconstruction images of CT and atlantoaxial instability does not appear in flexion/extension radiographs.

The long-term outcome of these patients is impressive. No postoperative neurological deficits and atlantoaxial instability, and no serious complications related to surgery, occurred in the case series; meanwhile a solid fixation and fusion without secondary kyphotic sagittal alignment of the subaxial spine were achieved, which does not depend on a solid external fixation.

In a word, preoperative thorough imaging evaluation and preparations, especially preoperative well reduction of the atlantoaxial articulation, should be required in order to prevent surgical complications. Under well preoperative preparations, bilateral C1–C2 transarticular screw and C1 laminar hook can provide a reliable fixation demanding for atlantoaxial instability. After then, large-scale prospective cohort studies might be conducted to further validate the efficiency and safety of bilateral C1–C2 transarticular screw and C1 laminar hook fixation and bone graft fusion.

References

1. Farey ID, Nadkarni S, Smith N. Modified Gallie technique versus transarticular screw fixation in C1–C2 fusion. Clin Orthop. 1999;359:126–35.
2. McAfee PCFI, Sutterlin CE, Gurr KR, et al. Device-related osteoporosis with spinal instrumentation. Spine. 1989;14:919–29.
3. Fielding JW, Hawkins RJ, Ratzan SA. Spine fusion for atlantoaxial instability. J Bone Joint Surg Am. 1976;58:400–7.
4. Melcher RP, Ruf M, Harms J. The direct posterior C1–C2 fusion technique with polyaxial-head screws. In: 28th Annual Meeting of the Cervical Spine Research Society, Charleston, South Carolina, 2000.
5. Magerl F, Seeman P-S. Stable posterior fusion of the atlas and axis by transarticular screw fixation. In: Kehr P, Werdner PA, editors. Cervical spine, vol. 1. New York: Springer-Verlag; 1987. p. 322–7.

6. Guo X, Ni B, Xie N, Lu X, Guo Q, Lu M. Bilateral C1-C2 transarticular screw and C1 laminar hook fixation and bone graft fusion for reducible atlantoaxial dislocation: a seven-year analysis of outcome. PLoS One. 2014;9(1):e87676. https://doi.org/10.1371/journal.pone.0087676.
7. Guo X, Ni B, Zhao W, Wang M, Zhou F, Li S, Ren Z. Biomechanical assessment of bilateral C1 laminar hook and C1-2 transarticular screws and bone graft for atlantoaxial instability. J Spinal Disord Tech. 2009;22(8):578–85.

Chapter 7
Clinical Anatomy and Image Measurements of Atlas and Axis in the Chinese Population and the Design of a Novel Hook + Screw Internal Fixation System

Jian Wang and Fei Chen

Abstract This chapter aims to measure linear and angular parameters of the atlas and axis in the Chinese population and provide a morphological basis for the design of the novel posterior atlantoaxial fixator. Thirty-five sets of normal adult dry atlas and axis vertebral samples and 40 sets of normal adult CT images of the upper cervical spine were measured. The parameters include posterior atlantal arch width, height, length, inside semi-diameter, outside semi-diameter, the transarticular screw path length, and the transarticular screw path angle in the transverse plane and in the sagittal plane.

7.1 Design of the Novel Posterior Atlantoaxial Fixator Composed of Bilateral Transarticular Screws and C1 Laminar Hooks

To reconstruct the stability of the atlas-axis complex, three-semi-diametral fixation is the best choice. Transarticular screw fixation combined with Gallie or Brooks technique and direct polyaxial screw fixation to the lateral masses of C1 or the pedicle of C2 can provide satisfactory atlantoaxial stability. However, the first has the risk of neural injury caused by the passage of sublaminar wires. The second needs high local surgical skill and has the risk of injury to the vertebral artery. A new technique for C1–C2 arthrodesis presented by Ni et al. [1] consists of a hook construct for the posterior arch of C1 that is rigidly attached to C1–C2 transarticular screws to form an instrument that combines anterior and posterior fixation in the same construct. This technique has the advantage over C1–C2 transarticular screw and Halifax clamps and provides excellent atlantoaxial stability that is equivalent to the Magerl-Brooks

J. Wang (✉)
Department of Orthopaedics, Pudong New Area People's Hospital, Shanghai, China
e-mail: doctoryangjian@126.com

F. Chen
Department of Orthopedics, Changzheng Hospital, Shanghai, China

B. Ni et al. (eds.), *Atlantoaxial Fixation Techniques*, Translational Medicine Research, https://doi.org/10.1007/978-981-10-7889-7_7

construct but can avoid the risks to placing cerclage wire under the C1–C2 arch. The currently available instruments have some problems and are not suitable for the Chinese population. A novel posterior atlantoaxial fixator composed of bilateral transarticular screws and C1 laminar hooks was designed to meet the technical and anatomical needs of the Chinese population. The novel posterior atlantoaxial fixator composed of bilateral C1 laminar hooks and C2 pedicle screws was also designed as an alternative choice when C1–C2 transarticular screw fixation is not feasible.

7.2 Clinical Anatomy and Image Measurements of the Atlas and Axis in the Chinese Population

Ni et al. [1] suggested a creative internal fixation with bilateral transarticular screws and C1 laminar hook. The three-point fixation streamline surgical technique reduces the risk of spinal cord injury and achieves sound fixation and fusion, which have been validated by preliminary studies. This chapter describes the development of the new internal fixation method in the Chinese population. Measuring 35 sets of dried atlas (C1) and axis (C2) specimens of normal adults and 40 sets of cervical CT materials of normal adults provided a reference for the designing of posterior cervical internal fixation devices.

7.2.1 Materials and Methods

7.2.1.1 Samples and Sampling

Thirty-five sets of dried C1–C2 bone specimens from normal adults were collected. We did not discriminate against any minority ethnic group, age group, or gender but did exclude specimens with deformities and defects. Pairs of C1–C2 came from one individual. Samples were provided by the Division of Anatomy of Second Military Medical University. Forty sets of cervical CT materials from normal adults (20 sets for each gender), with ages ranging from 20 to 70 years old, were collected. Samples with cervical pathology were excluded. CT materials were provided by the CT unit of the Shanghai Changzheng Hospital. Information on approval for this study from an ethics committee along with the full name of the committee and informed consent from participants should be provided as 35 sets of dried C1–C2 bone specimens from normal adults were collected in the study.

7.2.1.2 Anatomical Measurements

We conducted semi-diametral measurements on the dried specimens with local manufactured vernier calipers (accuracy, 0.02 mm). Measurements included the height and width of the posterior tubercle of the C1 posterior arch, the height and width of the posterior arch at 1 cm lateral to the C1 posterior tubercle (where the C1 laminar hook will be applied), and distal from the posterior tubercle to the vertebral artery groove (anterior-medial and posterior-lateral surfaces were measured, respectively, to find inner semi-diameter or outer semi-diameter).

7.2.1.3 Radiological Measurement

We used the Vitrea 2 version 3.5 platform for the semi-diametral measurement on the CT images (accuracy, 0.1 mm). Photoshop 7.0.1 was used as the measurement tool for the angular measurement (accuracy, 0.1°). The semi-diametral measurements included the height and width of the posterior arch at 1 cm lateral to the midline (where the C1 laminar hook will be applied) and the total length of the pathway of the simulated transarticular screws. Angular measurements included the angles between the pathway of the simulated transarticular screws and the transverse plane or sagittal plane (Figs. 7.1 and 7.2).

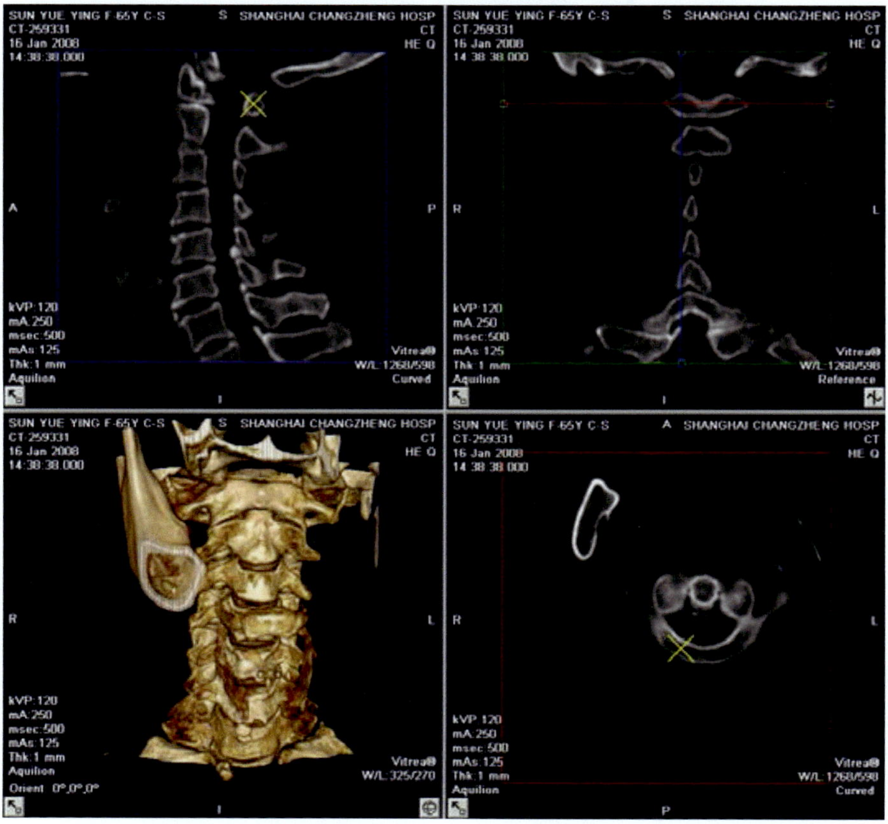

Fig. 7.1 Measurement and positioning of the C1 posterior arch and the pathway of the transarticular screw

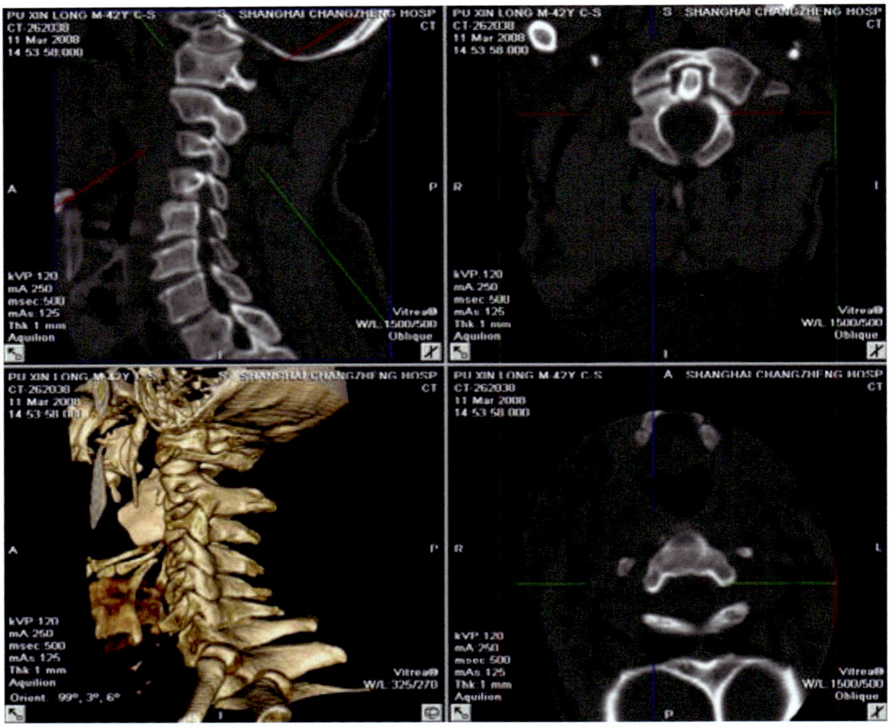

Fig. 7.1 (continued)

7.2.1.4 Statistics

All of the data was processed by SPSS15.0 statistics software. Anatomical and radiological measurements on each side of C1 and C2 were subjected to paired t-tests. Other relevant data from the anatomical and radiological measurements were subjected non-paired t-tests.

7.2.2 Results

7.2.2.1 Measurement of the C1 Posterior Arch

The height and width of the C1 posterior arch and inner/outer semi-diameter do not show a significant difference ($p > 0.05$) between the two sides; therefore, the bilateral data were pooled. For the dried specimens, the C1 posterior arch height was 9.52 ± 1.31 mm, the width was 6.30 ± 1.26 mm, the inner semi-diameter was 11.74 ± 2.47 mm, and outer semi-diameter was 20.49 ± 3.22 mm; for the CT images, the C1 height was 9.5 ± 1.6 mm and the width was 7.4 ± 1.3 mm.

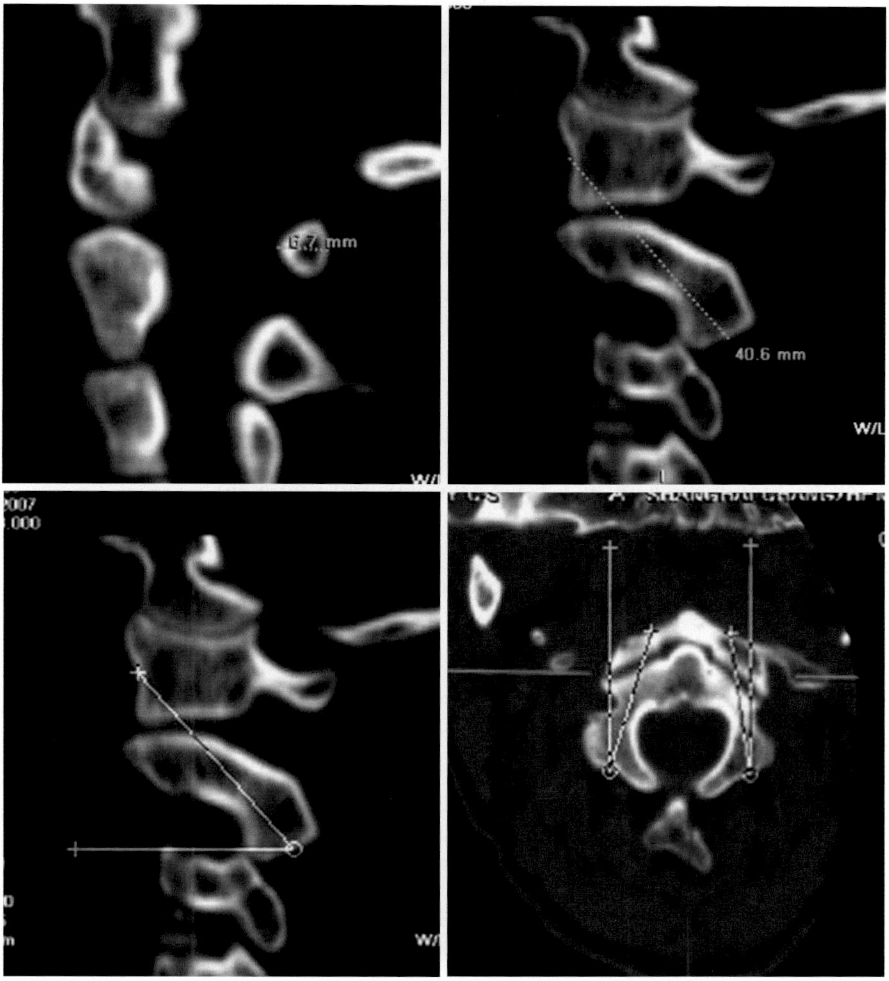

Fig. 7.2 Measurement of the C1 posterior arch and transarticular screw

Vitrea 2 version 3.5 platform is a very powerful platform that provides multi-plane reconstructions. It can create secondary cutting and reconstructions to create a cross-section of the spine at any position and with any angles.

The height and width of the C1 posterior arch were measured on the sagittal plane at 1 cm lateral to the posterior tubicle of C1, positioned on the transverse plane of C1. The subjects had a CT scan in the supine position. Thus, we kept the y-axis of the reconstructed sagittal view vertical during measurement so that the angle between the simulated pathway of the transarticular screw and the long axis of the body was applicable in real surgery. The midline was found by linking the C1 anterior tubercle, the center of the dents, and the center of the spinous process. The angle between the simulated transarticular screw pathway and midline was then measured (Fig. 7.2).

Measurements of the width of the C1 posterior arch from the dried specimens and radiology were significantly different ($p < 0.05$), but height measurements were not ($p > 0.05$) (Tables 7.1 and 7.2).

7.2.2.2 Measurement of C1–C2 Transarticular Screw

Bilateral data for the transarticular screw measurements showed no significant difference ($p > 0.05$); therefore, the bilateral data were pooled. The results showed a pathway length of 39.6 ± 3.4 mm, an angle to the cephalad of 52.0 ± 4.4°, and an angle to the midline of 9.1 ± 4.0° (Table 7.3).

7.2.3 Discussion

7.2.3.1 Significance of the C1–C2 Anatomy and Radiology

Most published data regarding the C1–C2 geometric measurements are based on the anatomical measurement of dry bone specimens, which is straightforward and reliable [2–9]. However, the availability of specimens is a problem. Meanwhile, the

Table 7.1 Anatomical measurements of dried specimens of C1 [$\bar{x} \pm s$, (min–max), $n = 35$, mm]

Location of measurement	Left	Right
Height of the C1 posterior arch	9.65 ± 1.40 (6.64–12.32)	9.39 ± 1.22 (7.20–11.74)
Width of the C1 posterior arch	6.32 ± 1.24 (4.16–8.70)	6.28 ± 1.30 (3.26–9.32)
Inner semi-diameter of the C1 posterior arch	11.78 ± 2.03 (7.28–16.10)	11.70 ± 2.86 (6.76–17.34)
Outer semi-diameter of the C1 posterior arch	20.37 ± 3.62 (11.90–27.80)	20.61 ± 3.00 (12.84–25.48)
Height of the posterior tubercle	10.29 ± 1.59 (6.66–12.94)	
Width of the posterior tubercle	7.44 ± 2.12 (4.06–11.80)	

Table 7.2 Anatomical measurement of 3D CT reconstruction of C1 [$\bar{x} \pm s$, (min–max), $n = 40$, mm]

Location of measurement	Left	Right
Height of the C1 posterior arch	9.6 ± 1.6 (7.3–12.6)	9.5 ± 1.5 (6.9–12.5)
Width of the C1 posterior arch	7.4 ± 1.4 (5.4–10.6)	7.3 ± 1.2 (5.7–9.9)

Table 7.3 C1–C2 transarticular measurements on 3D CT reconstruction [$\bar{x} \pm s$, (min–max), $n = 40$]

Measurement	Left	Right
Pathway length (mm)	39.8 ± 3 0.1 (36.5–48.0)	39.2 ± 3.6 (34.8–47.5)
Angle to the cephalad (°)	51.6 ± 3.8 (43.3–61.4)	52.3 ± 4.9 (38.3–60.2)
Angle to the midline (°)	8.9 ± 4.1 (2.5–14.9)	9.3 ± 4.0 (2.9–14.5)

irregular surface leads to a larger human error during measurement. In addition, dried specimens might have variation versus the in vivo condition because of dehydration or atrophy. However, it is more favorable to measure the height of the medial aspect of the C2 pedicle and the depth of the vertebral artery on dried specimens. In this case radiologically, it was difficult to pinpoint the position of the measurement.

Based on the comparison between measurement results of the C1 posterior arch from the two methods, we observed a significant difference in the width as determined by the two measurement methods, but not for the height. Measurement of the transarticular screw pathway based on CT 3D reconstruction and simulation was absolutely advantageous over the dried specimen method. Therefore, we adopted CT measurement of the C1 posterior arch and transarticular screw for subsequent analyses. Radiological measurement can be conducted on a large set of materials. The direct measurement of semi-diameters on CT 3D reconstruction software and determining and measuring the angles on Photoshop made the results more accurate. Meanwhile, the radiological data was obtained in in vivo conditions and is more relevant to clinical practice, making the results more indicative.

7.2.3.2 The Posterior Arch of C1

Understanding of the geometry of the C1 posterior arch is important to guide the exposure in the posterior approach. This study found that the inner semi-diameter was 11.74 ± 2.47 mm and outer semi-diameter was 20.49 ± 3.22 mm after pooling the bilateral data. Kaplan et al. [10] reported that the inner semi-diameter is 12–16 mm and outer semi-diameter is 22–28 mm. Li et al. [9] reported that the outer semi-diameter is 19.60 ± 3.58 mm for the left and 19.35 ± 3.14 mm for right and the inner semi-diameter is 11.57 ± 3.00 mm for the left and 11.42 ± 2.63 mm for the right. Zhu et al. [8] reported that the outer semi-diameter is 20.7 ± 3.05 mm for the left and 20.2 ± 2.77 mm for right and inner semi-diameter is 11.3 ± 2.98 mm for the left and 10.9 ± 2.56 mm for the right. Cao et al. [2] reported that the outer semi-diameter is 19.7 ± 4.4 mm for the left and 19.6 ± 4.4 mm for right; the inner semi-diameter is 11.4 ± 3.0 mm for the left and 11.5 ± 2.7 mm for the right. Thus, our results were close to other measurements reported from China.

To avoid injuring blood vessels and nerves in the vertebral artery groove, surgeons should be cautious when exposing or resecting the posterior arch. It is believed that exposure of the posterior arch should not be more than 10 mm. However, we have different considerations. The posterior arch is in a fan-shape with a certain curve. The vertebral artery groove is positioned from posterior-lateral to anterior-medial, and the inner semi-diameter is around 50% of that of the outer semi-diameter. Hence, if the spinal canal is not to be opened, when exposing the posterior arch, we can refer to the measurement of the outer semi-diameter, which is 20 mm. When exposing beyond 11 mm, we should be careful to avoid impinging on the neurovascular structure in the vertebral artery groove. If we are going to expose the posterior arch and enter into spinal canal, or resect the posterior arch, we should refer to the inner semi-diameter, which is no more than 11 mm. Note that some patients have a smooth posterior tubercle without obvious eminence, making it difficult to determine the position of posterior tubercle or the posterior arch. Given the condition of C1 rotation, it will be difficult to determine the left or right semi-diameter. We should be very careful when exposing the posterior arch to protect the vertebral artery.

In this study, the width of the C1 posterior arch was measured at 1 cm lateral to the midline of the C1 posterior tubercle, to which the laminar hook of C1 will be applied. The pooled data of the C1 posterior arch width from the dried specimen bilateral measurements was 6.30 ± 1.26 mm; and from the CT image, the width was 6.20 ± 1.16 mm. There is a significant difference between two methods. As CT assesses the in vivo condition, this study adopted the CT measurement results. Li et al. [9] reported width of 7.52 ± 2.50 mm for the left and 7.48 ± 2.48 mm for the right. Zhu et al. [8] reported a width of 6.7 ± 1.43 mm for the left and 6.5 ± 1.37 mm for the right. Cao et al. [2] reported a width of 6.3 ± 1.9 mm for the left and 6.5 ± 1.8 mm for the right. These Chinese authors all measured the width at the midpoint of the outer semi-diameter of the C1 posterior arch, which is equivalent to the area medial to the vertebral artery groove or 1 cm lateral to the midline of the C1 posterior tubercle where the C1 laminar hook is to be applied. This study adopted the CT measurement results. Their 95% confidence interval was 6.9–7.8 mm, with a minimum of 5.4 mm and a maximum of 10.6 mm. Our institute referred to this measurement when designing the width of the C1 laminar hook. The length of the hook also refers to the 9.5 ± 1.6 mm result measured by 3D CT in this study.

7.2.3.3 Transarticular Screw

Descriptions of the entry point for the C1–C2 transarticular screw are different; however, most of them are still within the medial 1/3 of the C2–C3 facet joint. Magerl et al. [5] took 3 mm superior to the inferior articular process and 2 mm lateral as the entry point. The trajectory is parallel to the sagittal plane and orients to the projection point of the posterior edge of the C1 anterior tubercle on the plane of trajectory. Paramore [11] took 4 mm cranial to the inferior edge of the C2–C3 facet joint and 2–3 mm lateral to the medial edge of the facet joint. The trajectory is parallel to the sagittal plane and orients to the projection of the midpoint of the C1 anterior tubercle on the plane of trajectory. Madawi et al. [12] took the most inferior aspect of the junction between the C2 pedicle and the inferior articular process. On the sagittal view, the trajectory should be somewhere between 0 and 15° to the medial and point to the tip of the C1 anterior tubercle. Marcotte et al. [13] took 2–3 mm lateral to the medial-inferior edge of the C2–C3 facet joint and 2–3 mm cranial as the entry point, with an angle between 0 and 10°. Chen et al. [6, 7] took the midpoint of the inferior edge of the C2 inferior articular process as the entry point. This study uses the Marcotte technique, which is 2–3 mm lateral and cranial to the medial-inferior edge of the C2–C3 facet joint. With this technique, the screw will perforate at the middle-superior edge of the C1 lateral mass with a bigger cephalad angle and a longer pathway to create a stronger fixation.

This study simulated a pathway of the transarticular screw and measured the length of the pathway and the angle to the cranial and the angle to the midline on a 3D CT reconstruction of C1–C2. The pooled data for the bilateral pathway length was 39.6 ± 3.4 mm. Chen et al. [6] performed the measurements on dried specimens: the left was 36.66 ± 2.75 mm and the right was 36.19 ± 2.91 mm. Ebraheim [14] measured the screw pathway on specimens and found that the best screw length is 38.1 ± 2.2 mm, independent of gender. The result of this study indicated a pathway length slightly longer than that shown in previous studies. This may be explained by the entry point option, loss of C1 height caused by dehydration, atrophy, and removal of joint cartilage. Excessive screw length might injure the sublingual nerve that runs anterior-lateral to the C1 lateral mass and the C1–C2 facet joint. A correct technique protects the sublingual nerve from injury. Intraoperatively screw length should be chosen individually. The drill bit should perforate the anterior cortex of the lateral mass for as long as possible. Screw lengths are chosen based on the direct measurement of the drill bit or by a depth gauge.

Software measurement of the simulated transarticular screw, after pooling of bilateral data, produced an angle to the cephalad of 52.0 ± 4.4° and angle to the midline of 9.1 ± 4.0°. Sha et al. [3] took 2 mm medial and superior to middle of the C2–C3 facet joint as the entry point. His measurement of the transarticular screw was angle to the cranial 39.2 ± 5.24° (left) and 9.3 ± 6.33° (right) and angle to the midline 5.67 ± 2.39° (left) and 6.68 ± 2.67° (right). The right side had a bigger angle toward the midline. Qu et al. [4] took the most inferior edge of the inferior articular process of C2 and the extension of the inferior edge of the C2 laminar as the entry point. The measurement of transarticular screw was angle to the cranial 51 ± 6° and angle to the midline as 12 ± 5° without significant difference between the left and right. Chen et al. [6] also reported measurements of the transarticular screw of the angle to the cephalad of 46.98 ± 4.02° (left) and 48.06 ± 5.12° (right) and angle to the midline, 12.53 ± 11.61° (left) and 13.65 ± 11.16° (right).

Madawi [12] suggested that the safety range of the angle to the midline of the screw is 0–14°. Solanki [15] analyzed the relationship between vertebral artery depth and angle of the screw using computer-assisted design (CAD). Solanki suggested that when the length of the pedicle is 30 mm, every 0.5 mm increment in the depth of the vertebral artery groove requires an additional 1° of screw angle. There is a linear relationship between the angle of the screw and pedicle width. The author suggested that the screw of 3.5 mm diameter should have an additional 7° on top of the cephalad angle of the pedicle. The variance of measurement is explained by the different entry points. There is a big variance of angle to the midline of the transarticular screw in our study, 2.5–14.9°, which indicated that we need to pay attention to the variance between pedicles.

7.2.3.4 Safety of the C1–C2 Transarticular Screw

The pathway of the transarticular screw is lateral to the spinal cord, medial to the vertebral artery, and posterior to the sublingual nerve. As the spinal canal is relatively big at C1, the risk of spinal cord injury is minor. Vertebral artery impingement is the major risk for transarticular screws. Gebhard et al. [16] reported that up to 15% of C1–C2 transarticular screws are malpositioned. Wright et al. [17] collected materials of 1318 cases. Thirty-one (2.4%) of them had documented vertebral artery injury. Twenty-three (1.7%) had suspicious vertebral artery injury. Madawi [12, 18] reported that five out of 61 cases (8.2%) had vertebral artery injury.

The suitability of the transarticular screw for C1–C2 fixation depends on the width and height of the bone for screw to purchase. The variation of the vertebral artery groove has a direct impact on the width and height of the C2 pedicle. Some authors believe that among cases with an indication for C1–C2 fusion, 18–23% are not suitable for transarticular screw fixation because they have variation of the vertebral artery at least on one side.

Madawi [12, 18] measured 25 independent axials and found that 20% of pedicles were not suitable for transarticular fixation. Cao et al. [2] measured the width of the middle part of the pedicles and found that 72% of them were wider than 5 mm and could accommodate a 3.5 mm Magerl screw. Kong et al. [19] believed that measurement of the medial height at 2.5 cm to the superior edge of the pedicle was able to predict the impact of a small pedicle on screw fixation. He found that 21.5% of the specimens were not suitable for posterior C1–C2 transarticular screw fixation. Igarashi [20] measured the anatomical parameters of the pedicles of C2 and the vertebral artery recess and found that 20% of pedicles of C2 were smaller than the screw diameter (3.5 mm) with huge variance and asymmetry. He suggested that there was a higher risk of vertebral artery injury when the width or height was less than 3.5 mm.

Foreign studies commonly state that 20% of cases are not suitable for a 3.5 mm screw. This study suggested that although some cases may have a small pars on one or both sides, the drill bit or screw might crack the lateral cortex and compress the vertebral artery, it does not necessarily lead to compromised blood supply of the vertebrobasilar artery system and create symptoms.

To ere on the side of caution, preoperative radiological investigation of the pars of C2 pedicles should be conducted. In case of severe deformity of the pars, alternative methods should be used. Thorough preoperative radiological investigations and preparation, skillful surgical technique, and sound intraoperative X-ray control can reduce the incidence of vertebral artery injury. Fuji et al. [21] reported 111 transarticular screw fixations from 56 patients; 95.5% of the screws were in a good position. No vertebral artery injury was reported in that study.

Marcotte et al. [13] suggested that C1 and C2 should be reduced adequately to ensure a good screw pathway. Minor dislocation can be fixed by adjusting the screw trajectory. Kong et al. [19] suggested that transarticular screw fixation will work if the C1 anterior translation is no more than 8.93 ± 4.17 mm. However, this estimate was based on the screw trajectory in a single line. Considering the diameter of the screw, we should make adjustments during the procedure. To reduce the possibility of vertebral artery injury, we should achieve as much preoperative reduction as possible preoperatively.

7.2.4 Conclusion

Based on the result of this study and a literature review, the width of the C1 posterior arch of the Chinese population is around 7.4 ± 1.3 mm. When exposing the posterior arch and entering the spinal canal, or resecting the posterior arch, the scope of exposure should not be beyond the inner semi-diameter of 11.74 ± 2.47 mm. The length of the transarticular screw pathway is around 39.6 ± 3.4 mm. The screw should be around 52.0 ± 4.4° to the cranial and 9.1 ± 4.0° to the midline. The C1 and C2 of most Chinese people are suitable for bilateral atlas laminar hook and C1–C2 transarticular screw fixation. As C2 pedicles have significant individual variance, we should investigate the pedicles preoperatively using parasagittal plane thin-slice CT and plan the surgery individually. The surgery should be monitored by X-ray control or navigation. For patients who are not eligible for transarticular screw fixation, C2 pedicle screws plus C1 laminar hook, C2 pedicles screws plus C1 lateral mass screws, or pedicle screws are alternatives.

Good surgical technique deserves relevant internal fixation devices. Under the guidance of bilateral C1 laminar hook and C1–C2 transarticular screw techniques, and based on the data from experimental measurement and literature review, we designed and produced a novel posterior internal fixation device for C1 and C2 and studied its biomechanical performance.

7.3 Design of a Novel Bilateral C1–C2 Transarticular Screw and C1 Laminar Hook Internal Fixation System

7.3.1 Design Software and Materials

We used the CAX'A Design System developed by Beijing Beihang Haier Software Co. (provided by Shanghai Surgical Instruments Factory). The implant material was Ti-6Al-4V (TC4), which is the most widely used titanium alloy in clinical practice. TC4 enjoys the best flexibility and stiffness. Its stiffness is 60% that of stainless steel. Its density is around 4.5–19.3 g/cm^3, which is similar to human bone. Meanwhile it has sound biochemical compatibility; i.e., it is free of cytotoxicity, carcinogenicity, tissue irritation, and immune reaction and has good mechanical features, good resistance to erosion, fatigue, friction, and sound smoothness. It does not get magnetized nor affects postoperative magnetic resonance imaging (MRI) examination (Table 7.4).

Table 7.4 Physical parameters of titanium alloy for the novel C1–C2 posterior internal fixation system

Tensile strength (MPa)	Yield strength (MPa)	Fatigue strength (MPa)	Impact toughness (kg m/cm^2)	Brinell hardness (HB)	Young's elastic modulus (kMPa)	Elongation (%)
1055	995	450	3.1	324	110	7.5

The manufacturing process includes wire cutting, machine tools, drilling, milling for teeth, polishing, dry spraying, and passivation. The manufacturing equipment includes a wire-cutting machine, general machine tools, a milling and drilling machine, a polishing machine, and a blasting machine (all provided by Shanghai Surgical Instruments Factory).

7.3.2 Geometry Design and Specification of the Bilateral C1–C2 Transarticular Screw and C1 Laminar Hook Internal Fixation System

The fixation system comprises two parts: a screw and a hook. Graphic design, prototyping, trial use on specimens, and amendment have been respectively conducted before finalization. (See Fig. 7.3 for the master design).

7.3.2.1 The Hook

The C1 laminar hook has an adjustable joint and is composed of the laminar hook and an adjustable joint and rod. The laminar hook comprises a hook that extends into a ring end. There is a groove on the top of the hook to accommodate the jaw of the compression forceps. The under surface of the hook has teeth to reduce slippage. The adjustable joint links the hook with the rod. It is composed of a rotation axis and cap. The outer diameter of the main body of the rotational axis is compatible

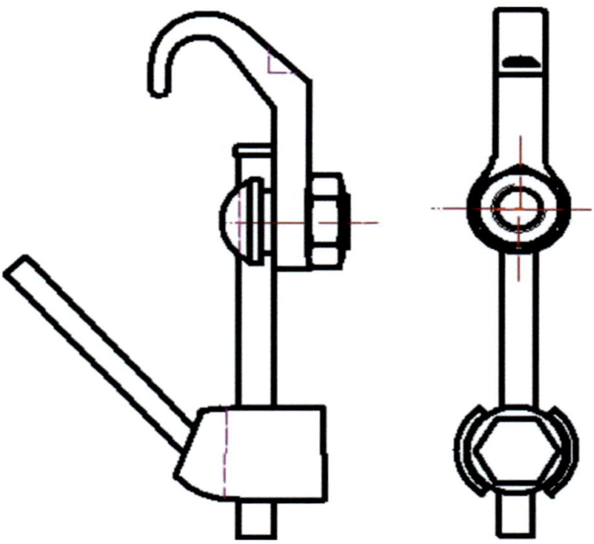

Fig. 7.3 Design of the novel bilateral C1–C2 transarticular screw and C1 laminar hook internal fixation

with the inner diameter of the ring. One end of the axis has a hole for the rod to go through, while the opposite end has thread for the cap to seat on. The outer diameter of the rod is compatible with the inner diameter of the hold on the axis. The end of the rod has a collar to stop the rod from moving. The end of the rod also has teeth to match the teeth of the ring so that the two parts can be stably fixed at different angles.

For assembly, the rod is inserted into the hole in the axis. The ring end of the hook is put onto the axis; the cap is seated on the threaded axis and turned tightly to form a C1 laminar hook with a joint.

7.3.2.2 The Screw

The C2 polyaxial screw is composed of a screw body, screw head, and locking cap. The head is cannulated with a 50° inclining bottom. The screw body is connected with the screw hole of the head. There are two U-shape openings on each side of the head. The width of the U opening is compatible with the connecting rod of the laminar hook. The screw head has an inner thread that matches the thread of the locking cap. The locking cap is cannulated with a hexagonal cross-section of the cannulation. A hexagonal screwdriver of compatible size should be used to lock the cap. As the bottom of the screw head has an inclination of 45°, the screw can have a bigger cephalad angulation to fulfill the angulation requirement of the transarticular screw (Fig. 7.4).

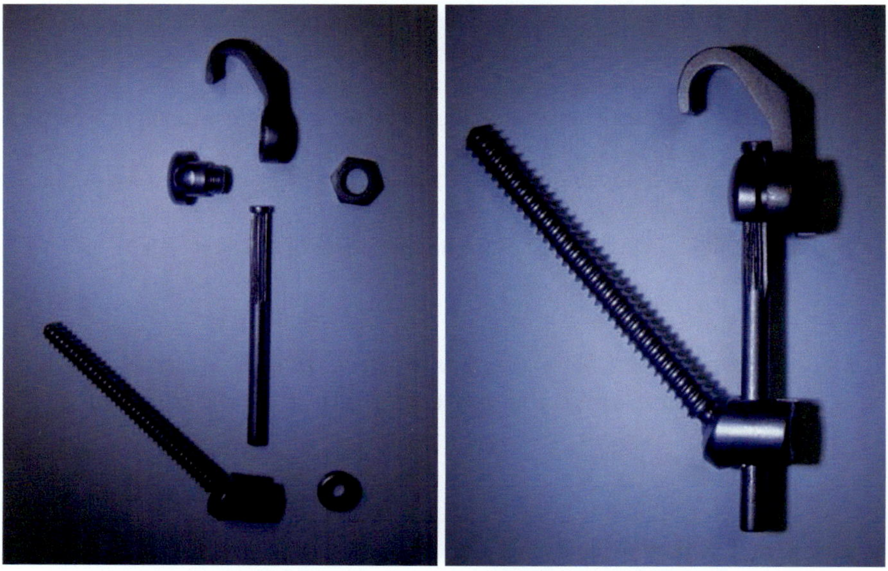

Fig. 7.4 Parts and assembly of the novel C1–C2 posterior fixation system

7.3.2.3 Specification

The laminar hook is 4.5 mm in width, 3 mm in thickness in the body, and 2 mm to 1 mm tapering from the curve to the tip. There are a couple of inner diameter options, such as 2.8 mm and 3.0 mm. The rod is 40 mm in length and 3 mm in outer diameter. The body of the polyaxial screw has two diameters, 3.5 mm and 4.0 mm, and the length varies from 24 mm to 44 mm, with 2 mm increments. The inner diameter of the screw head is compatible with the outer diameter, which is 7.8 mm.

7.3.3 Features of the Design and Functions

1. With the joint of the C1 laminar hook, the angle between the hook and the rod is adjustable. To make assembly easier and have a good fit between the hook and the C1 posterior arch, the contact surface is enlarged and with less stress concentration. Hooks with different sizes can fit with individual C1 posterior arches of Chinese patients. It is not necessary to remove the bone to fit the size of the hook.
2. There are teeth on the curved surface of the hook to prevent slippage. The end of the rod has teeth along the longitudinal axis. These teeth match the teeth on the ring of the hook so that the system can be locked at different angles and is very stable.
3. The bottom of screw head inclines at 50°, providing a larger cephalad angulation for the screw body. It can fulfill the requirement of big angulation between the transarticular screw and its head. It also makes the connection between the screw head and body easy, while reducing the stress concentration around the junction.
4. Cortical screws of 3.5 and 4 mm in diameter are mechanically strong enough and fulfill the anatomical requirements of most patients.
5. The compression forceps groove on the top of the hook allows compression with forceps to increase the fusion rate.
6. The rotation axis of the joint of the C1 laminar hook can extend for easy connection of a cross-link, which can stop the bone graft from migrating, resulting in higher stability and leaving room for improvement of the next step.

7.3.4 Assembly and Implantation of the Novel Bilateral C1–C2 Transarticular Screw and C1 Laminar Hook Internal Fixation System

The operation should be monitored by C-arm X-ray control. The entry point of the screw is at the intersection point of the sagittal line, which passes the pars crest and the inferior edge of the C2 laminar. Find the medial edge of the inferior articular process of C2 and go 2 mm superior and 2 mm lateral. Open the cortex of the entry point with a manual drill bit. The drill bit should advance on the sagittal plane along the medial aspect of the C2 pedicle pars, penetrate the posterior part of the C1–C2 facet joint, and enter into the lateral mass of C1. Caution should be taken to avoid penetrating the cortex and damaging the vertebral artery laterally and spinal cord medially.

Use a ball-tip probe to explore the depth of the pathway and bony tunnel to make sure it is not outside the bone. Choose a screw of the appropriate length. After tapping the pathway, insert the polyaxial cortical screw into the pathway carefully. After insertion, use the same technique to insert the contralateral screw. Turn the screw head to make a 50° angle toward the cephalad so that the screw head remains level. Afterward, adjust the joint of the C1 laminar hook to the appropriate angle, apply temporal fixation, and apply the hook onto the posterior arch of C1. Insert the rod into the U-shape opening of the polyaxial transarticular screw. Insert the lock cap and pre-tighten.

Collect a T-shape graft with the cortical bone on two sides from the right posterior superior iliac spine. Clean up the grafting bed. Use a high-speed burr to decorticate the C1 posterior arch surface and the inferior and superior aspects of the C2 laminar. Insert the trimmed graft into the space between the C1 posterior arch, the C2 spinous process, and the bilateral rods. Simultaneously compress the internal fixation system with the compress forceps to secure the graft and make a good fit of the C1 hook with the posterior arch. Final tighten the joint of the hook and locking cap of the transarticular screw. Thus, through the C1 laminar, the rod, and the ipsilateral C1–C2 transarticular screw, the C1 posterior arch is fixed with a graft and the ipsilateral C2 laminar. Pack bone debris on the exposed bone surface and decorticated C1–C2 facet joints. The unstable C1–C2 joint now is grafted, compressed, and fixed (Figs. 7.5, 7.6, and 7.7).

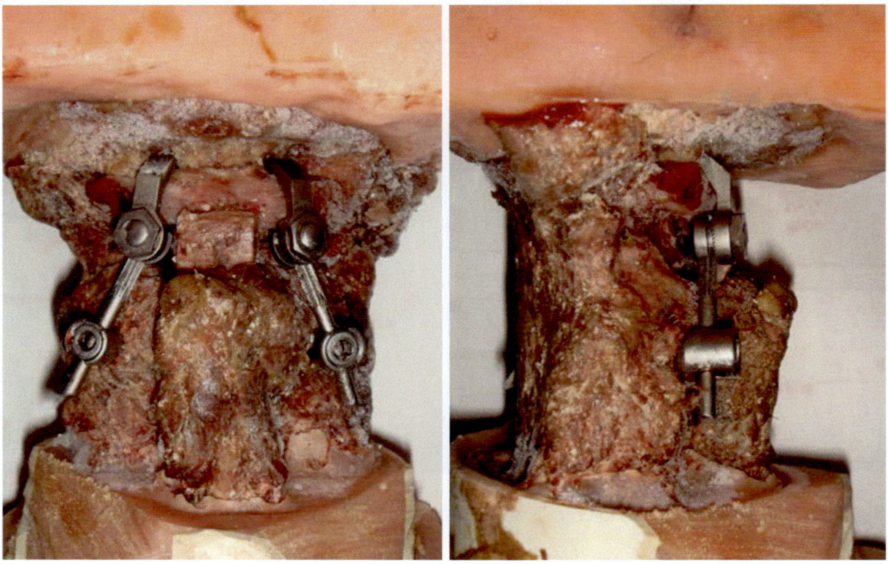

Fig. 7.5 Posterior and lateral view of the novel C1–C2 posterior internal fixation system implanted

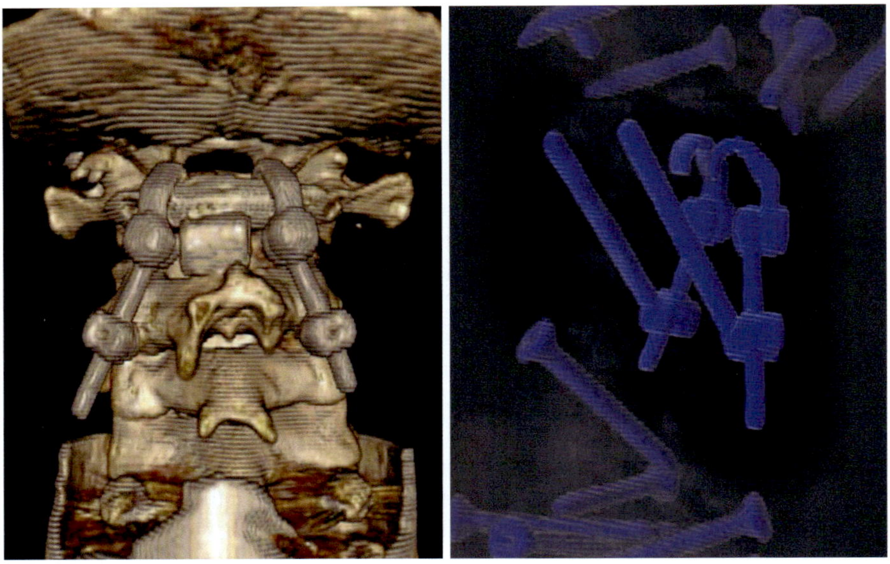

Fig. 7.6 Posterior and oblique view of the novel C1–C2 posterior internal fixation system with CT reconstruction

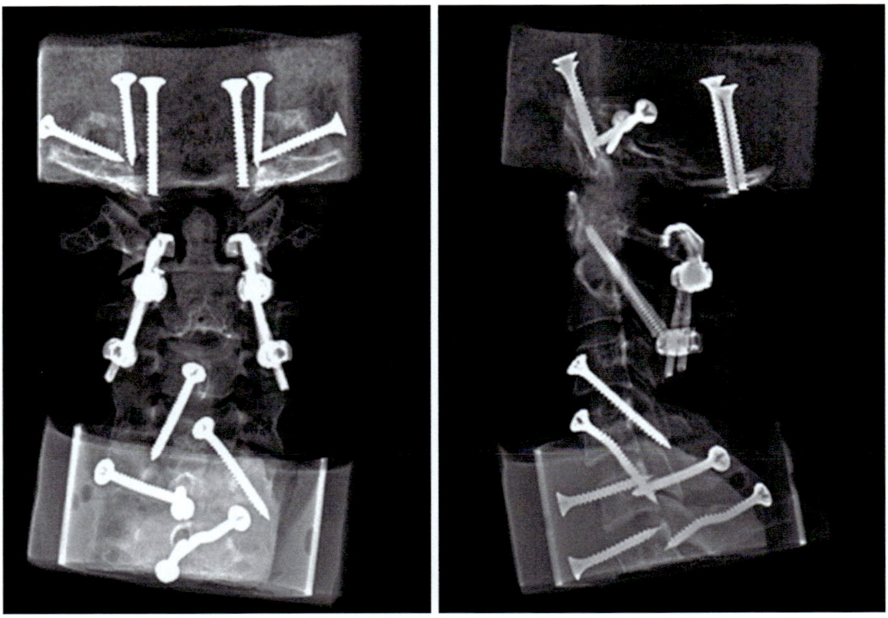

Fig. 7.7 Anteroposterior and lateral view of the implanted novel C1–C2 posterior internal fixation system under X-ray

7.4 Novel Bilateral Pedicle Screws and C1 Laminar Hook Internal Fixation System

To solve the problem of C2 anatomy variation, for example, the deep vertebral artery groove, of some patients who are not suitable for transarticular screws, we designed a bilateral C2 pedicle and a C1 laminar hook internal fixation system. This system comprises a hook, rod, and screw. The difference between this system and the bilateral C1–C2 transarticular screw and C1 laminar hook system is that the screw is shorter and is used for C2 pedicles. The rods are shorter, while the C1 laminar hooks are the same. The surgical technique is almost identical to the bilateral C1–C2 transarticular screw and C1 laminar hook system. The only difference is that it uses the relatively easier C2 pedicle screw. Although this internal fixation is not a three-point fixation and its biomechanical stability must be lower than that of the C1–C2 transarticular screw and C1 laminar hook, it is still useful for patients with a low requirement for stability. It can replace transarticular screws on one or both sides. Being assisted by reliable postoperative external immobilization, it can achieve ideal fixation. This internal fixation system enriches surgical techniques of atlantoaxial displacement and expands surgical indications.

References

1. Ni B, Chen H, Guo X, et al. Bilateral C1–2 transarticular screws and atlas hooks fixation technique. Zhonghua Wai Ke Za Zhi. 2005;43:1358–9. (Chinese Language)
2. Cao Z, Zhong S, Xu D. Atlantaoaxial anatomic measurement and its clinical signification. Zhong Guo Linchuang Jie Pou Za Zhi. 2000;18(4):299–301. (Chinese Language)
3. Sha Y, Zhang S, Liu Z, et al. Atlantoaxial anatomic measurement of posterior C1–2 transarticular screws. Zhongguo Linchuang Jie Pou Za Zhi. 2002;20(3):172–5. (Chinese Language)
4. Qu D, Jin D, Zhu Z, et al. Chinese anatomic measurement of atlantoaxial transarticular screws. Zhongguo Linchuang Jie Pou Za Zhi. 2000;7(11):1117–9.
5. Magerl F, Seeman PS. Stable posterior fusion of the atlas and axis by transarticular screw fixatior. In: Kehr P, Weidner A, editors. Cervical spine. 4th ed. New York: Springer Verlag; 1985. p. 322–7.
6. Chen ZH, Lun-Hong YU, Huang JF, et al. Anatomic study of radiologic parameters about new location mark in the posterior atlanto-axial transarticular screw fixation. Chin J Clin Anat. 2005;23(5):463–6. (Chinese Language)
7. Chen Z, Cai X, Huang J, et al. Applied anatomic and clinical studies on posterior atlantoaxial facet screw fixation. Chin J Exp Surg. 2005;22:159–60. (Chinese Language)
8. Zhu H, Jia L, Sun Q, et al. Measurement of atlas and its clinical significance. Chin J Anat. 1997;20(6):517–20. (Chinese Language)
9. Li QH, Liu YB, Sheng DH, et al. Applied anatomical study of atlas. J Gannan Med Univ. 2003;23(4):363–7. (Chinese Language)
10. Kaplan EB. Surgical approaches to the neck. Cervical spine and upper extremity. London: Saunders; 1966. p. 246.

11. Paramore CG, Dickman CA, Sonntag VKH. The anatomical suitabilityof the C1-2 complex for transarticular screw fixatior. J Neurosurg. 1996;85:221–4.
12. Madawi AA, Casey TH, Solanki GA, et al. Radiologieal and anatomical evaluation of the atlantoaxial transarticttlar screw fixation technique. J Neurosurg. 1997;86:961–8.
13. Mareotte P, Dickman CA, So nntag VKH, et al. Posterior at1antoaxial facet screw fixation. Neurosurg. 1993;79:234–7.
14. Ebraheim NA, Misson JR, Xu R, et al. The optimal transarticular C1-2 Screw length and the location of the hypoglossal nerve. Surg Neurol. 2000;53(3):208–10.
15. Solanki GA, Crockard HA. Peroperative determination of safe superior transarticular screw trajectory through the lateral mass. Spine. 1999;24:1477–82.
16. Gebhard JS, Schimmer RC, Jeannerel B. Safty and accuracy of transarticular screw fixation C1–C2 using an aiming device: an anatomic study. Spine. 1998;23:2185–9.
17. Wright NW, Lauryssen C. Vertebral artery injury in C1-2 transarticular screw fixation: results of survey of the AANS/CNS section on disorders of the spine and peripheral nerves. J Neurosurg. 1998;88(4):634–40.
18. Madawi A, Solanki G, Casey AT, et al. Variation of the groove in the axis vertebra for the vertebral artery: implications for instrumentation. J Bone Joint Surg Br. 1997;79:820–3.
19. Kong QY, Jia-Shun LI, Jia LS. Anatomic measurements of the transarticular screw fixation of the atlantoaxial. Orthop J China. 2002;11(10):1328–30.
20. Igarashi T, Kikuchi S, Sato K, et al. Anatomic study of the axis for surgical planning of transarticular screw fixation. Clin Orthop Relat Res. 2003;408:162–6.
21. Fuji T, Oda T, Kato Y, et al. Accuracy of atlantoaxial transarticular screw fixation. Spine. 2000;25(14):1760–4.

Chapter 8
Limitations of TA + Hook Technique

Songkai Li and Fengjin Zhou

Abstract Although the previous section showed that the TA + Hook technique is an excellent technique that provided more rigid stabilization and higher fusion rates for the treatment of atlantoaxial instability, this technique still has some limitations, including potential injury to the vertebral arteries, complete preoperation reduction of the atlantoaxial joint, and unsuitability for patients with fracture or congenital absence of the posterior arch of atlas. Based on the anatomical study of the atlanto-axial lateral masses, a lateral mass fusion cage was designed. The biomechanical study demonstrated that the C1 + C2 + Cage technique, when the posterior lamina of the atlas is absent or removed for decompression, might be a viable option for the stabilization of the atlantoaxial complex.

On the basis of the transarticular screw technique of Magerl, Ni et al. [1] introduced the C1–C2 transarticular screw supplemental C1 laminar hook fixation (TA + Hook), which is connected with posterior rods combined with autologous iliac crest bone grafts wedged between the lamina of C1 and the spinous process of C2, developing a modified three-point fixation technique. In a biomechanical study, Guo et al. demonstrated that a bilateral TA + Hook can provide significantly stronger biomechanical stability than that obtained by two-point system [2], as well as inducing higher rates of fusion and satisfactory clinical results [1, 3–7]. Although the TA + Hook fixation provides satisfactory biomechanical results and clinical outcomes, there are still some patients who are precluded from this technique because of anatomical variations in the atlantoaxial complex.

S. Li (✉)
Department of Orthopedics, Lanzhou General Hospital, Lanzhou, Gansu, China

F. Zhou
Department of Spinal Surgery, Xi'an Zhongde Orthopedics Hospital, Xi'an, Shanxi, China

B. Ni et al. (eds.), *Atlantoaxial Fixation Techniques*, Translational Medicine Research, https://doi.org/10.1007/978-981-10-7889-7_8

8.1 The Potential Risk of Vertebral Arteries Injury

It is known to all that there are risks of vertebral artery (VA) injuries with the technique of C1–C2 transarticular screw. Several anatomical or radiological studies of the atlantoaxial region have demonstrated that up to 20% of patients may not be suitable candidates for transarticular screw fixation on at least one side because of a high-riding transverse foramen [8–10]. Madawi et al. [11], in their retrospective review of 61 patients who underwent transarticular screw fixation, reported five cases involving a VA injury. Gluf et al. [12] reported 6 VA injuries (1.7%) in 5 patients in 191 patients in whom 353 consecutive transarticular screws were placed, and 1 bilateral VA injury resulted in the patient's death. Wright and Lauryssen [13] surveyed 847 active members of the American Association of Neurological Surgeons/Congress of Neurological Surgeons (AANS/CNS) regarding the risk of VA injury in transarticular screw fixation. They demonstrated that 31 (2.4%) of 1318 patients were known to have VA injury and an additional 23 (1.7%) had suspected injuries, with a 0.2% incidence of subsequent neurological deficit and a 0.1% mortality rate. However, Grob et al. [14] reported no damage to the VA after review of a series of 161 consecutive patients operated by several different surgeons at four different Swiss hospitals. Stillerman and Wilson [15] also reported no incidence of VA damage among 22 cases of posterior transarticular screw fixation. Although the rates of vertebral artery injury seem to be very low, it is mandatory to appreciate this catastrophic complication when this technique is performed. The variation of anatomic course of the vertebral artery through C2 should be scrutinized carefully preoperative using a computed tomography (CT) reconstructions in the sagittal and coronal planes to determine whether there is a high-riding VA under the superior articular facet of the axis. Some authors defined the high-riding VA based on CT reconstruction, which is a simple and widely accepted method of evaluation [11, 16, 17]. They adopted Bloch et al.'s [18] definition of the high-riding VA: an internal height less than 2 mm, an isthmus height and width less than 5 mm, or both. However, the isthmus height and width are more important because the screw goes through the isthmus itself regardless of the internal height. Therefore, some patients, who had an isthmic height and width of C2 are less than 5 mm in CT reconstruction, may have been more prone to injure the VA during the placement of the C1–C2 transarticular screw with a diameter of 3.5 mm. If C2 cannot safely to insert the screw, other techniques, such as C1 lateral mass/C2 pedicle screw technique or C1 lateral mass/C2 translaminar screw technique, should be applicable to patients to stabilize the atlantoaxial joint. If a suspected VA injury has occurred during placement of the first transarticular screw, the screw should be placed to tamponade bleeding, and placement of a second screw should not be attempted to obviate bilateral VA injury. In addition, for some patients with excessive cervicothoracic kyphosis and obesity, this technique would be impossible due to the acute angle of approach needed for screw placement.

8.2 The Importance of Complete Reduction of the Atlantoaxial Joint During Operation

Intraoperatively, a satisfactory reduction of a dislocation of the atlantoaxial joint is essential. If there is any subluxation, anteriorly or posteriorly dislocation, the points of screw intersection should be altered, thus affecting the evaluation of the risk and the guidance of the screw trajectory. Madawi et al. [11] emphasized the importance of complete reduction of the atlantoaxial joint before passage of the screw. They noted nine cases of screw malposition in 14 cases with incomplete reduction, and all five VA injuries were associated with incomplete reduction. Thus, complete reduction of the atlantoaxial articulation is necessary prior to placement of the screw. Persistent anterior dislocation of C1 on C2 might be reduced by pushing anteriorly on the spinous process of C2 and pulling posteriorly by a wire placed around the posterior arch of C1. Alternatively, persistent posterior dislocation of C1 on C2 may be reduced by pulling posteriorly on the spinous process of C2 with a Kocher clamp and pushing anteriorly on the intact posterior arch of C1 with a thumb [19]. This procedure decreases the incidence of VA injury by bringing the VA into a more normal anatomical position.

8.3 A Lateral Mass Fusion Cage with a C1–C2 Pedicle Fixation Technique for the Treatment of Atlantoaxial Instability with Congenital Absence or Fracture of Posterior Arch of C1

In the TA + Hook technique, an intact posterior arch of C1 is necessary for hooks to compress a bone graft between the C1 posterior arch and the C2 spinous process for fusion. However, in certain patients, such as those with congenital anomalies or bone loss from previous surgery, the posterior arch of C1 is deficient or fractured, which makes it impossible to use the posterior arch of C1 to place the graft. In this situation, the TA + Hook technique is not possible, and an alternative fusion technique is necessary to treat the atlantoaxial instability.

Various methods have been used to achieve atlantoaxial fusion when the posterior arch of the atlas is absent or removed for decompression, and a Gallie fixation is impossible. Extending the instrumentation and fusion to the occiput is advocated frequently, particularly when non-unions are involved [20, 21]. Although it bridges the C1 segment to achieve fusion from the occiput to C2, it also sacrifices the normal occiput–C1 motion, which can be an important component of the patient's flexion and extension motion, and is especially important in the initiation of swallowing.

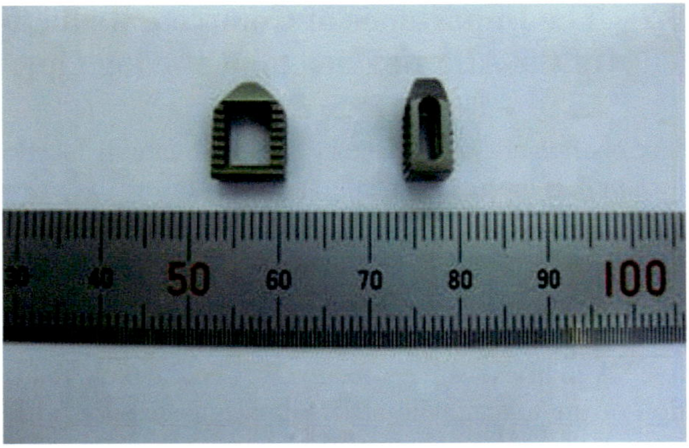

Fig. 8.1 Superior and lateral view of the cages

The recent popularity of the use of interbody fusion cages fused to the spine suggests that atlantoaxial lateral mass fusion using a cage could be an alternative treatment for atlantoaxial stabilization when previous surgeries have failed or when regional anatomical variation makes posterior atlantoaxial fusion impossible. If successful, this approach would allow rigid C1–C2 fixation without the need to extend the instrumentation and fusion to the occiput and would preserve the normal occiput–C1 motion.

To preserve this important motion segment, we designed a lateral mass fusion cage based on an anatomical study of the atlantoaxial lateral masses [22]. The anatomical data indicated that three sizes of cage were feasible: 11/8 mm, 12/9 mm, and 13/10 mm (length/width) and 3.5, 4, and 4.5 mm in height (Fig. 8.1). Various other sizes are available to meet individual requirements using different standards. A cadaver model was used to evaluate and compare the stability of the fusion cage combined with the C1 + C2 pedicle screw technique with that of the Magerl + Gallie and C1 + C2 pedicle screw method (Fig. 8.2). No statistically significant differences were found among the three stabilization methods. The C1 + C2 + Cage technique could provide other fusion spots for atlantoaxial stabilization with similar stabilities to current methods. Thus, when the posterior lamina of the atlas is absent or removed for decompression and a Gallie fixation is impossible, the C1 + C2 + Cage technique might be a viable alternate to stabilization of the atlantoaxial joint.

8.4 Limitations Associated with Instruments

The instruments that are applied currently in the clinic can have some problems and are not suitable for the Chinese population. For example, the laminar hooks were made originally for the thoracic laminar and are not particularly suitable for the atlas posterior arch, making the hook and the screw difficult to connect. A novel posterior atlantoaxial fixator comprising bilateral transarticular screws and C1 laminar hooks was designed to overcome the technical challenge and conform to the anatomical properties of the Chinese population. The biomechanical study showed that the novel fixator provided similar stability to other fixation techniques [23].

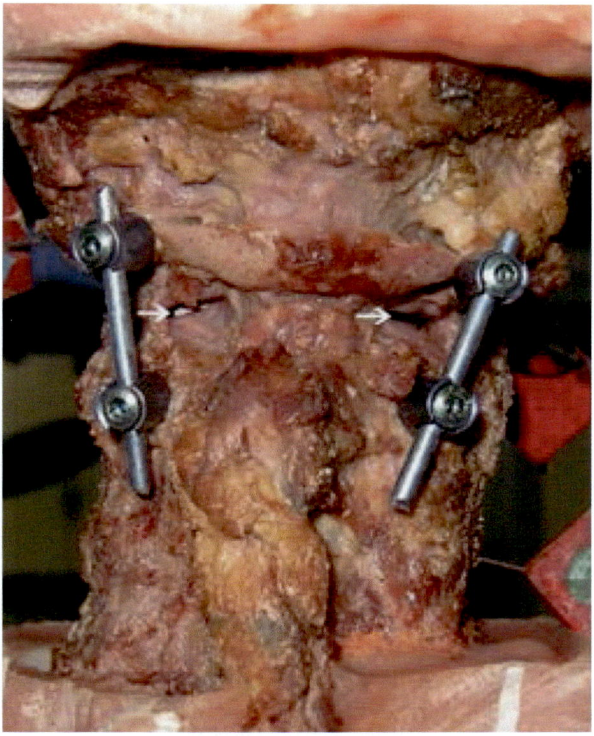

Fig. 8.2 A cadaveric specimen after the C1 + C2 + Cage (arrow) technique

References

1. Ni B, Chen HJ, Guo X, Tao CS. Bilateral C1-C2 transarticular screw and C1 laminar hook fixation. Chin J Surg. 2005;43:1358–9.
2. Guo X, Ni B, Zhao WD, Wang MF, Zhou FJ, Li SK, Ren ZW. Biomechanical assessment of bilateral C1 laminar hook and C1-2 transarticular screws and bone graft for atlantoaxial instability. J Spinal Disord Tech. 2009;22:578–85.
3. Guo QF, Liu J, Ni B, Lu XH, Zhou FJ. C2 laminar screw and C1-2 transarticular screw combined with C1 laminar hooks for atlantoaxial instability with unilateral vertebral artery injury. Arch Orthop Trauma Surg. 2011;131:1207–10.
4. Guo X, Ni B, Wang MF, Wang J, Li SK, Zhou FJ. Bilateral atlas laminar hook combined with transarticular screw fixation for an unstable bursting atlantal fracture. Arch Orthop Trauma Surg. 2009;129:1203–9.
5. Guo X, Ni B, Xie N, Lu XH, Guo QF, Lu M. Bilateral C1-C2 transarticular screw and C1 laminar hook fixation and bone graft fusion for reducible atlantoaxial dislocation: a seven-year analysis of outcome. PLoS One. 2014;9:e87676.
6. Ni B, Guo X, Xie N, Li SK, Zhou FJ, Zhang F, Liu Q. C1-2 transarticular screws combined with C1 laminar hooks fixation: a modified posterior atlantoaxial fixation technique and outcome in 72 patients. Eur Spine J. 2013;22:260–7.
7. Ni B, Guo X, Xie N, Lu XH, Yuan W, Li SK, Zhou FJ, Zhu ZC. Bilateral atlantoaxial transarticular screws and atlas laminar hooks fixation for pediatric atlantoaxial instability. Spine (Phila Pa 1976). 2010;35:E1367–72.
8. Farey ID, Nadkarni S, Smith N. Modified Gallie technique versus transarticular screw fixation in C1-C2 fusion. Clin Orthop Relat Res. 1999;359:126–35.

9. Madawi AA, Solanki GA, Casey AT, Crockard HA. Variation of the groove in the axis vertebra for the vertebral artery. Implications for instrumentation. J Bone Joint Surg Br. 1997;79:820–3.
10. Goel A, Gupta S. Vertebral artery injury with transarticular screws. J Neurosurg. 1999;90:376–7.
11. Madawi AA, Casey AT, Solanki GA, Tuite G, Veres R, Crockard HA. Radiological and anatomical evaluation of the atlantoaxial transarticular screw fixation technique. J Neurosurg. 1997;86:961–8.
12. Gluf WM, Schmidt MH, Apfelbaum RI. Atlantoaxial transarticular screw fixation: a review of surgical indications, fusion rate, complications, and lessons learned in 191 adult patients. J Neurosurg Spine. 2005;2:155–63.
13. Wright NM, Lauryssen C. Vertebral artery injury in C1-2 transarticular screw fixation: results of a survey of the AANS/CNS section on disorders of the spine and peripheral nerves. American Association of Neurological Surgeons/Congress of Neurological Surgeons. J Neurosurg. 1998;88:634–40.
14. Grob D, Bremerich FH, Dvorak J, Mannion AF. Transarticular screw fixation for osteoarthritis of the atlanto axial segment. Eur Spine J. 2006;15:283–91.
15. Stillerman CB, Wilson JA. Atlanto-axial stabilization with posterior transarticular screw fixation: technical description and report of 22 cases. Neurosurgery. 1993;32:948-54; discussion 954–5.
16. Dickman CA, Sonntag VK. Posterior C1-C2 transarticular screw fixation for atlantoaxial arthrodesis. Neurosurgery. 1998;43:275–80;discussion 280–1.
17. Papagelopoulos PJ, Currier BL, Hokari Y, Neale PG, Zhao C, Berglund LJ, Larson DR, An KN. Biomechanical comparison of C1-C2 posterior arthrodesis techniques. Spine (Phila Pa 1976). 2007;32:E363–70.
18. Bloch O, Holly LT, Park J, Obasi C, Kim K, Johnson JP. Effect of frameless stereotaxy on the accuracy of C1–2 transarticular screw placement. J Neurosurg. 2001;95:74–9.
19. Jeanneret B, Magerl F. Primary posterior fusion C1/2 in odontoid fractures: indications, technique, and results of transarticular screw fixation. J Spinal Disord. 1992;5:464–75.
20. Dickman CA, Sonntag VK. Surgical management of atlantoaxial nonunions. J Neurosurg. 1995;83:248–53.
21. Nakagawa T, Yone K, Sakou T, Yanase M. Occipitocervical fusion with C1 laminectomy in children. Spine (Phila Pa 1976). 1997;22:1209–14.
22. Li SK, Ni B, Xie N, Wang MF, Guo X, Zhang F, Wang J, Zhao WD. Biomechanical evaluation of an atlantoaxial lateral mass fusion cage with C1–C2 pedicle fixation. Spine (Phila Pa 1976). 2010;35:E624–32.
23. Wang MF. Design and biomechanical study of the novel posterior atlantoaxial fixator composed of bilateral transarticular screws and Cl laminar hooks. Shanghai: Second Military Medical University; 2008.

Chapter 9
Using the Principle of Translational Medicine to Improve the Posterior "Hook-Screw" Atlantoaxial Fixation

Jun Yang and Qunfeng Guo

Abstract This chapter describes the basic principle of translational medicine and its application to the posterior "hook-nail" atlantoaxial fixation technique.

Translational medicine evolved from translational studies in the 1990s. It is characterized by basic clinical research being carried out in a multidisciplinary cross-cooperation mode, so that the research findings can be applied clinically and quickly to achieve "experimental-to-clinical" translation. New problems identified during clinical application are fed back to the laboratory to provide new research ideas. Thus, mutual translation between basic research and clinical application is realized so that both sides are closely associated to form a bi-directional, open, and successive development cycle. Its core concept and final objective are to build an effective link between the researchers engaged in basic scientific studies and the doctors who know the patients' needs, allowing transfer of the findings of basic research into actual disease prevention, diagnosis, treatment, and post-assessment services for patients, thus overcoming diseases and promoting human health.

The surgical treatment of the atlantoaxial instability currently consists of open reduction and partial fixture fusion. The therapeutic principle is to retain as much movement as possible via short-segment fusion. Therefore, atlantoaxial fusion has become a major treatment method and consists of anterior and posterior fusions [1], of which the latter are used more frequently in the clinic. The traditional treatment methods include wire binding (including the Gallie and Brooks methods), Apofix and Halifax lamina hooking, Magerl screwing, and other improved methods. Gallie, Brooks, and similar methods comprise single-point fixation, which can control the atlantoaxial sagittal bend/stretch movement to a certain extent but cannot control the axial rotation between the atlantoaxial vertebrae. Therefore, the bone-grafting fusion rate is relatively low and is always prone to failure of internal

J. Yang · Q. Guo (✉)
Department of Orthopedics, Changzheng Hospital, Shanghai, China
e-mail: guoqunfeng83@163.com

B. Ni et al. (eds.), *Atlantoaxial Fixation Techniques*, Translational Medicine Research, https://doi.org/10.1007/978-981-10-7889-7_9

fixation. Moreover, cables going through the vertebral lamina can easily cause injury to spinal nerves during surgery. As the fixing strength is limited, the immediate stability cannot be achieved after surgery, but auxiliary fixing may be required in the long term.

The Apofix and Halifax lamina hooking methods have one fixing point, but only the under-lamina operating procedure is simplified, and a larger hook is designed, which may easily press on the vertebral canal, which could result in new spinal compression to produce a mal-reduced atlantoaxial dislocation.

The Magerl screwing technique, also called joint space screw, offers two-point fixation and can control the axial rotation between the atlantoaxial vertebrae. A biodynamic study indicated that the joint space screw can provide relatively strong immediate stability and the bone-grafting fusion rate was 86.9–100%. However, as the sagittal bend/stretch movement is controlled poorly, simple screwing results in an internal fixation failure rate as high as 50% [2]. Madawi [3] reported a 4% internal fixing failure ratio. Therefore, many scholars have combined the joint space screw and the Gallie or Brooks method to improve the bone-grafting fusion rate, which is an ideal three-point fixing method and could control flexion-and-extension and horizontal axial rotational movements between atlantoaxial vertebrae effectively; however, it still requires cabling under the laminas, possibly injuring spinal nerves. In addition, fixing failure and bone-graft non-fusion are still possibilities. Klimo et al. [4] used the joint space screws and a lasso technique to treat nine atlantoaxial instability cases, among which screws were ruptured in two cases. Cornefjord et al. used the Olerud Cervical Fixation System (formed by connecting the arcus posterior the atlas claw with the joint space screws via a connecting rod) to treat 26 cases of atlantoaxial instability, among which fusion failure occurred in three cases [5].

Considering the increasing surgical cases of clinical atlantoaxial dislocation, the limitations of various clinical internal fixation methods, the wide and effective application of the posterior screw-rod system, the features of the small thoracic vertebrae hook, and the combined features of the screw-rod system, Professor Ni Bin united the available clinical internal fixing methods to make use of the strong two-point stability of Magerl screwing method and the three-point stability achieved by Apofix's upper hooking structure [6]. Ni used a fine thoracic vertebral hook to reduce the hook's possible occupation of the vertebral canal, and adopted the screw (hook)-rod connection, which is a frequently used posterior connection method for the spine, to achieve a built-up connection, such that the multiway pre-bending plasticity of the connecting rod could achieve the complex posterior connection of the atlantoaxial vertebra effectively. The internal fixing method simultaneously realized three-point fixing of Magerl screwing and Gallie or Brooks methods, enhanced stability, improved the bone-grafting fusion rate, and simplified the operating procedures, achieving a satisfactory outcome during preliminary clinical application. However, the new internal fixing method lacks experimental support and verification. Thus, the problems proposed clinically should be verified during the basic research according to the concept of the translational medicine.

For this reason, under the leadership of Professor Ni Bin, a series of relevant experimental studies have been carried out. Biodynamic studies related to the hook-nail system proved that the hook-nail system has powerful stability in all active directions (such as fore and aft flexion, extension, lateral flexion, and horizontal rotation), which was higher than the stability achieved by current internal fixing methods or their combinations [7]. The results indicated that this internal fixation system was well designed. Finite element analysis also confirmed the reasonable mechanical distribution of the method, without obvious stress concentration [8]. Clinical practices were carried out in parallel, with the bulk of cases showing outstanding curative effects, and the indications of this new fixation technique have been widened gradually [9].

While satisfactory results have been obtained, some treatment failures have occurred. Good reduction and high arch of the vertebral artery could not be achieved under anesthesia in some cases, and thus the screw could not be inserted into the joint space, which was a new problem that appeared during clinical application. In such cases, an improved hook-nail system was proposed, the C2 pedicle screw (or isthmus screw) associated with a C1 lamina hook screw-rod system. This new method could be substitute for the preferred method [6]. Although it may be considered as a single-point fixing method, its clinical bone-grafting fusion rate was very high. In terms of vertebral artery injury during surgery or special dissection variation, the combined fixing method could guarantee smooth surgical performance and reliability of the fixture [10]. Relevant basic research will be carried to corroborate the clinical findings.

References

1. Melcher RP, Ruf M, Harms J. The direct posterior C1-C2 fusion technique with polyaxial-head screws. In: 28th annual meeting of the Cervical Spine Research Society. Charleston, SC; 2000. p. 120–6.
2. Magerl F, Seeman P-S. Stable posterior fusion of the atlas and axis by transarticular screw fixation. In: Kehr P, Werdner PA, editors. Cervical spine, vol. 1. New York: Springer; 1987. p. 322–7.
3. Madawi AA, Casey AT, Solanki GA, Tuite G, Veres R, Crockard HA. Radiological and anatomical evaluation of the atlantoaxial transarticular screw fixation technique. J Neurosurg. 1997;86(6):961–8.
4. Klimo P Jr, Kan P, Rao G, Apfelbaum R, Brockmeyer D. Os odontoideum: presentation, diagnosis, and treatment in a series of 78 patients. J Neurosurg Spine. 2008;9(4):332–42.
5. Cornefjord M, Henriques T, Alemany M, Olerud C. Posterior atlanto-axial fusion with the Olerud Cervical Fixation System for odontoid fractures and C1-C2 instability in rheumatoid arthritis. Eur Spine J. 2003;12(1):91–6.
6. Ni B, Zhu Z, Zhou F, Guo Q, Yang J, Liu J, Wang F. Bilateral C1 laminar hooks combined with C2 pedicle screws fixation for treatment of C1-C2 instability not suitable for placement of transarticular screws. Eur Spine J. 2010;19(8):1378–82.
7. Guo X, Ni B, Zhao W, Wang M, Zhou F, Li S, Ren Z. Biomechanical assessment of bilateral C1 laminar hook and C1–2 transarticular screws and bone graft for atlantoaxial instability. J Spinal Disord Tech. 2009;22(8):578–85.

8. Chen J, Zhou F, Ni B, Guo Q, Guan H, Xu T, Liu Q. New posterior atlantoaxial restricted non-fusion fixation for atlantoaxial instability: a biomechanical study. Neurosurgery. 2016;78(5):735–41.
9. Guo X, Xie N, Lu X, Guo Q, Deng Y, Ni B. One-step reduction and fixation applying trans-posterior arch lateral mass screw of C1 combined with pedicle screw of C2 and rod system for pediatric acute atlantoaxial rotatory subluxation with injury of transverse ligament. Spine (Phila Pa 1976). 2015;40(5):E272–8.
10. Yang J, Ni B, Yan W, Zhou F, Chen J. Post atlantoaxial fusion for unilateral cleft of atlas posterior arch associated with os odontoideum: case report and technique note. Eur Spine J. 2011;20(Suppl 2):S284–8.

Chapter 10
Atlantoaxial Personalized Fixations Including Transarticular Screws + Atlas Hooks

Peng Zhang

Abstract Different fusion techniques are used to treat atlantoaxial instability, including posterior wiring, interlaminar clamps, C1–C2 TAS, the Harms technique, and crossing C2 ILS technique. However, variants of the VA is relatively common; therefore, there is an urgent need for personalized fixation combinations. Unilateral TAS and contralateral C2PS combined with bilateral C1 LMS and C2ILS and TAS combined with bilateral C1LH have been used as alternatives to traditional techniques. The biomechanics of these two fixation combinations have been confirmed. In addition, a combination of bilateral C1LH and C2ILS is considered a good choice in terms of biomechanics and VA safety.

Abbreviations

C1LH	C1 laminar hook
C1LMS	C1 lateral mass screw
C2ILS	C2 intralaminar screw
C2PS	C2 pedicle screw
CVJ	Craniovertebral junction
CT	Computed tomography
ROM	Range of motion
TAS	Transarticular screw
VA	Vertebral artery

The atlantoaxial complex, which accounts for 50% of rotation and 12% of flexion/extension of the cervical spine [1], can be unstable secondary to a range of disorders, including congenital, neoplastic, traumatic, and degenerative pathologies.

P. Zhang
Department of Orthopedics, Changzheng Hospital, Shanghai, China

B. Ni et al. (eds.), *Atlantoaxial Fixation Techniques*, Translational Medicine Research, https://doi.org/10.1007/978-981-10-7889-7_10

However, the choice of an ideal fixation technique is a challenge. An optimal fixation should not only provide good stability but also should minimize the risk of spinal cord and VA injury. During the last few decades, there has been rapid development in atlantoaxial stabilization techniques, including posterior wiring, interlaminar clamps, C1–C2 TAS, Harms technique, and the C2ILS technique. Among them, stabilization techniques using wiring [2, 3] and interlaminar clamps [4, 5] are easier to achieve. However, they do not provide sufficient immobilization across the C1–C2 complex. Furthermore, wiring techniques may suffer frequent neurological problems caused by sublaminar wire passage. In contrast, the TAS technique achieves a biomechanically stiffer C1–C2 arthrodesis and a clinically significant improvement in the fusion rate. Nevertheless, the TAS technique is associated with the serious complication of VA injury, which is not inherent in the former techniques [6–8]. The Harms technique is another method of C1–C2 arthrodesis that can reduce the risk of VA injury [9]. Biomechanical studies of this technique, Melcher et al. [10] and Richter et al. [8] found that it provided more stability than TAS. Conversely, a previous study confirmed that it is effective in immobilizing the C1–C2 complex but offers less stability slightly than the TAS technique [11]. Kuroki et al. [12] reported that with unilateral fixation, TAS provided significant stability in the axial rotation only, whereas Harms technique was effective in all modes, except extension. And with bilateral fixation, Harms technique was superior to TAS in flexion and extension. However, placement of the C2PS can be problematic because of the aberrant course of the VA and the fact that 20% axis vertebrae have effective pedicle diameters <3.5 mm [13]. As a modification, the crossing C2ILS technique [14], with comparable biomechanics with Harms technique [15], can avoid the path of the VA in the C2 segment; however, it still leaves the VA in the C1 segment exposed to injury owing to C1LMS misplacement [16] or an abnormal VA course in the posterior arch of C1 [17].

Previous studies have shown anomalies of the VA at the extra- and intraosseous regions of the CVJ [18–24]. There are two representative anomalies of the extraosseous course of the VA: fenestration and persistent first intersegmental artery. In the former, the VA duplicated after emerging from the C2 transverse foramen; one branch enters the spinal canal between C1 and C2, and the other courses normally, passing through the C1 transverse foramen and entering the spinal canal at the cranial side of the C1 posterior arch [18, 19]. In the latter, the VA enters the spinal canal at the caudal portion of the C1 posterior arch after emerging from the C2 transverse foramen, without passing through the C1 transverse foramen [20, 21]. Studies have also demonstrated congenital variations in size of the VAs, ranging from asymmetry of both VAs to severe unilateral VA hypoplasia. More frequently, the left VA diameter is larger than the right. In a postmortem study, Krayenbuhl and Yasargil [25] found that 42% was larger on the left, 32% was larger on the right, and 26% was approximately equal bilaterally. In an angiographic study, Kazui et al. [26] found that the left was wider in 61%, the right was wider in 33%, and both VAs were equal in only 6%. Also in duplex ultrasound studies, Bartels et al. [27] and Yuan et al. [28] found that the average VA diameter was more often larger on the left side than on the right. In good agreement with previous studies, the blood flow volume assessed by duplex ultrasound demonstrated higher blood flow volume in the left VA than in the right [29, 30]. When an intraosseous VA is located anomalously too medially, too posteriorly, and/or too high, it is described as "high-riding" [20]. Yamazaki et al. [31] analyzed 100 consecutive patients who underwent CVJ instrumentation surgery since July 1998 using three-dimensional computed tomographic angiography (3D CTA) and found that the frequencies of fenestration, persistent first intersegmental artery, high-riding VA, and side-to-side asymmetry in the atlantoaxial subluxation group were 3, 14, 34, and 19%. In addition, the frequency of an abnormal VA at the extra- and intraosseous regions is increased when patients have atlantoaxial subluxation and congenital skeletal anomaly at the CVJ. Furthermore, 43.04% adolescent population is found with the concomitant of the ponticulus posticus, which is a bony bridge arising from the posterior portion of the superior articular process and the posterolateral portion of the superior margin of the posterior arch of the atlas that encircles the vertebral artery completely or partially.

In light of these variants in the VA, the development of a personalized fixation combination is imperative as an alternative to current fixation techniques. For patients whose C2 pedicle screw placement on one side would not be possible because of an aberrant VA, osseous structures, or unilateral VA occlusion, Matsubara et al. [32] and Du et al. [33] applied hybrid fixation techniques comprising a unilateral translaminar screw, a contralateral C2 pedicle screw, and bilateral C1LMS as an alternative or salvage. The biomechanics of this fixation combination were verified by Gorek et al. [34] However, VA in the C1 segment is still exposed to injury from C1LMS misplacement [16] or an abnormal VA course in the posterior arch of C1 [17]. Furthermore, for similar patient, Sugimoto et al. [35] and Guo et al. [36] applied C2ILS and TAS combined with a bilateral atlas hook as an alternative. The biomechanics of this combination were confirmed by Zhang et al. [11], who reported that bilateral atlas hook and C2ILS was superior to bilateral TAS fixation in terms of biomechanics and VA safety.

Considering the unique anatomy of the atlantoaxial complex, there is a need for surgeons to apply personalized fixation combinations instead of the current standard fixation techniques, which should have comparable stability and minimized risk of VA and spinal cord injury. We propose that priority should be given to the safety of the spinal cord and VA, proactively. For side-to-side asymmetry VA, ensuring the dominant VA is imperative, considering that the circle of Willis functions as an anastomosis and can offer a potential shunt under abnormal conditions [37]. Following this, stability of fixation should be emphasized.

References

1. White AA 3rd, Panjabi MM. The clinical biomechanics of the occipitoatlantoaxial complex. Orthop Clin North Am. 1978;9:867–78.
2. Brooks AL, Jenkins EB. Atlanto-axial arthrodesis by the wedge compression method. J Bone Joint Surg Am. 1978;60:279–84.
3. McGraw RW, Rusch RM. Atlanto-axial arthrodesis. J Bone Joint Surg (Br). 1973;55:482–9.

4. Cybulski GR, Stone JL, Crowell RM, et al. Use of Halifax interlaminar clamps for posterior C1-C2 arthrodesis. Neurosurgery. 1988;22:429–31.
5. Moskovich R, Crockard HA. Atlantoaxial arthrodesis using interlaminar clamps. An improved technique. Spine (Phila Pa 1976). 1992;17:261–7.
6. Dickman CA, Sonntag VK. Posterior C1-C2 transarticular screw fixation for atlantoaxial arthrodesis. Neurosurgery. 1998;43:275–80; discussion 80-1.
7. Solanki GA, Crockard HA. Peroperative determination of safe superior transarticular screw trajectory through the lateral mass. Spine (Phila Pa 1976). 1999;24:1477–82.
8. Richter M, Schmidt R, Claes L, et al. Posterior atlantoaxial fixation: biomechanical in vitro comparison of six different techniques. Spine (Phila Pa 1976). 2002;27:1724–32.
9. Harms J, Melcher RP. Posterior C1-C2 fusion with polyaxial screw and rod fixation. Spine (Phila Pa 1976). 2001;26:2467–71.
10. Melcher RP, Puttlitz CM, Kleinstueck FS, et al. Biomechanical testing of posterior atlantoaxial fixation techniques. Spine (Phila Pa 1976). 2002;27:2435–40.
11. Zhang P, Liu Q, Xu T, et al. Biomechanical study of 3 atlantoaxial proactive vertebral artery injury prevention fixation combinations. World Neurosurg. 2016;93:293–8.
12. Kuroki H, Rengachary SS, Goel VK, et al. Biomechanical comparison of two stabilization techniques of the atlantoaxial joints: transarticular screw fixation versus screw and rod fixation. Neurosurgery. 2005;56:151–9; discussion 151-9.
13. Abou Madawi A, Solanki G, Casey AT, et al. Variation of the groove in the axis vertebra for the vertebral artery. Implications for instrumentation. J Bone Joint Surg (Br). 1997;79:820–3.
14. Wright NM. Posterior C2 fixation using bilateral, crossing C2 laminar screws: case series and technical note. J Spinal Disord Tech. 2004;17:158–62.
15. Claybrooks R, Kayanja M, Milks R, et al. Atlantoaxial fusion: a biomechanical analysis of two C1-C2 fusion techniques. Spine J. 2007;7:682–8.
16. Tan M, Wang H, Wang Y, et al. Morphometric evaluation of screw fixation in atlas via posterior arch and lateral mass. Spine (Phila Pa 1976). 2003;28:888–95.
17. Huang MJ, Glaser JA. Complete arcuate foramen precluding C1 lateral mass screw fixation in a patient with rheumatoid arthritis: case report. Iowa Orthop J. 2003;23:96–9.
18. Yamazaki M, Okawa A, Aramomi MA, et al. Fenestration of vertebral artery at the craniovertebral junction in Down syndrome: a case report. Spine (Phila Pa 1976). 2004;29:E551–4.
19. Yamazaki M, Koda M, Yoneda M, et al. Anomalous vertebral artery at the craniovertebral junction in a patient with Down syndrome. Case report. J Neurosurg Spine. 2004;1:338–41.
20. Yamazaki M, Koda M, Aramomi MA, et al. Anomalous vertebral artery at the extraosseous and intraosseous regions of the craniovertebral junction: analysis by three-dimensional computed tomography angiography. Spine (Phila Pa 1976). 2005;30:2452–7.
21. Yamazaki M, Okawa A, Hashimoto M, et al. Abnormal course of the vertebral artery at the craniovertebral junction in patients with Down syndrome visualized by three-dimensional CT angiography. Neuroradiology. 2008;50:485–90.
22. Takahashi M, Kawanami H, Watanabe N, et al. Fenestration of the extra-cranial vertebral artery. Radiology. 1970;96:359–60.
23. Kowada M, Yamaguchi K, Takahashi H. Fenestration of the vertebral artery with a review of 23 cases in Japan. Radiology. 1972;103:343–6.
24. Carella A, Lamberti P, Federico F, et al. Double fenestration of the extracranial vertebral artery. Neuroradiology. 1978;15:193–4.
25. Krayenbuhl H, Yasargil MG. [The vascular diseases in the region of the basilar & vertebral arteries; an anatomopathological, clinical & neuroradiological study]. Fortschr Geb Rontgenstr Nuklearmed. 1957;87:1–170.
26. Kazui S, Kuriyama Y, Naritomi H, et al. Estimation of vertebral arterial asymmetry by computed tomography. Neuroradiology. 1989;31:237–9.
27. Bartels E, Fuchs HH, Flugel KA. Duplex ultrasonography of vertebral arteries: examination, technique, normal values, and clinical applications. Angiology. 1992;43:169–80.
28. Yuan RY, Yip PK, Liu HM, et al. The value of duplex and continuous wave Doppler sonography for evaluation of the extracranial vertebral arteries: a prospective comparison with angiography. Zhonghua Yi Xue Za Zhi. 1994;53:42–8.

29. Schoning M, Walter J, Scheel P. Estimation of cerebral blood flow through color duplex sonography of the carotid and vertebral arteries in healthy adults. Stroke. 1994;25:17–22.
30. Seidel E, Eicke BM, Tettenborn B, et al. Reference values for vertebral artery flow volume by duplex sonography in young and elderly adults. Stroke. 1999;30:2692–6.
31. Yamazaki M, Okawa A, Furuya T, et al. Anomalous vertebral arteries in the extra- and intraosseous regions of the craniovertebral junction visualized by 3-dimensional computed tomographic angiography: analysis of 100 consecutive surgical cases and review of the literature. Spine (Phila Pa 1976). 2012;37:E1389–97.
32. Matsubara T, Mizutani J, Fukuoka M, et al. Safe atlantoaxial fixation using a laminar screw (intralaminar screw) in a patient with unilateral occlusion of vertebral artery: case report. Spine (Phila Pa 1976). 2007;32:E30–3.
33. D S, Ni B, Lu X, et al. Application of unilateral C2 translaminar screw in the treatment for atlantoaxial instability as an alternative or salvage of pedicle screw fixation. World Neurosurg. 2017;97:86.
34. Gorek J, Acaroglu E, Berven S, et al. Constructs incorporating intralaminar C2 screws provide rigid stability for atlantoaxial fixation. Spine (Phila Pa 1976). 2005;30:1513–8.
35. Sugimoto Y, Tanaka M, Nakanishi K, et al. Safety of atlantoaxial fusion using laminar and transarticular screws combined with an atlas hook in a patient with unilateral vertebral artery occlusion (case report). Arch Orthop Trauma Surg. 2009;129:25–7.
36. Guo Q, Liu J, Ni B, et al. C2 laminar screw and C1-2 transarticular screw combined with C1 laminar hooks for atlantoaxial instability with unilateral vertebral artery injury. Arch Orthop Trauma Surg. 2011;131:1207–10.
37. Kamath S. Observations on the length and diameter of vessels forming the circle of Willis. J Anat. 1981;133:419–23.

Part III

Development and Related Basic Research of a New Posterior Atlantoaxial Fixation Technique

Abstract

This section focuses on the basic study of new posterior atlantoaxial fixation techniques. The first chapter describes an integrated C1 laminar hook applied in atlantoaxial fusion which is modified based on previous combination of C1 hook and C1-2 transarticular screws or C2 pedicle screws systems. The design process, manufacture, and the biomechanical tests of the new integrated C1 laminar hook are presented. The second chapter describes a new C1 long-tail reduction lateral mass screw which can facilitate the reduction of atlantoaxial dislocation combined with C2 pedicle screw. The design process, manufacture, and reduction procedure are described in detail.

Chapter 11
Modification of Posterior Integrated C1 Laminar Hooks Applied in Atlantoaxial Fusion

Ming Lu and Ning Xie

Abstract Every posterior C1–C2 fixation system has advantages and disadvantages. This chapter describes the drawbacks of the combination of a C1 hook and C1–C2 transarticular screws or C2 pedicle screws, and modification of the posterior integrated C1 laminar hooks applied in atlantoaxial fusion.

The atlantoaxial joint connects the cervical spine and cranial skull and is known for its unique anatomy and for adjoining the cervical spinal cord and vertebral arteries. The unique anatomy results in unique functions; however, tumors, anomalies, inflammation, and degeneration are the main causes of instability of the atlantoaxial joint. Atlantoaxial instability is a challenge for spinal surgeons and can result in compression of spinal cord and/or vital vessels. If untreated, atlantoaxial instability could lead to paresis or even sudden death. Surgical intervention to create atlantoaxial fusion is the treatment of choice of atlantoaxial instability. There are anterior and posterior approaches for atlantoaxial arthrodesis surgery, among which anterior dens screws fixation, anterior transarticular fixation, and anterior transoral atlantoaxial reduction plate (TARP) fixation are used commonly. However, they are not feasible for most of patients because of the complicated regional anatomy and limited indications. Therefore, the posterior approach is more popular. Posterior atlantoaxial fusion surgery has moved from wiring fixation (Gallie technique and Brooks technique), posterior laminar hook fixation (Halifax, Apofix), C1–C2 transarticular screw, to posterior C1–C2 screw-rod fixation. The wiring technique is a one-point fixation and maintains flexion-extension but performs poorly for bilateral bending or rotation, and the fusion failure rates are high [1]. Recently the C1–C2

M. Lu
Department of Orthopedics, Changzheng Hospital, Shanghai, China

N. Xie (✉)
Department of Spine Surgery, Shanghai Tongji Hospital, Tongji University, Shanghai, China
e-mail: drnxie@163.com

B. Ni et al. (eds.), *Atlantoaxial Fixation Techniques*, Translational Medicine Research, https://doi.org/10.1007/978-981-10-7889-7_11

transarticular screw fixation and posterior C1–C2 screw-rod fixation techniques have become the main methods to treat atlantoaxial instability. Previous biomechanical and clinical studies confirmed that such fixations stabilize the atlantoaxial joint with high fusion rates [2]. However, bilateral C1–C2 transarticular fixation is a two-point fixation and performs poorly for flexion-extension stability. If combined with posterior wiring and structural graft, it achieves satisfactory motion restriction in all directions because of three-point fixation. A biomechanical study showed that bilateral C1–C2 transarticular screw combined with posterior wiring fixation plus bone fusion provides superior biomechanical strength [3]. This technique has been proved biomechanically to be the gold standard treatment for atlantoaxial instability.

However, there is substantial risk of spinal cord injury introduced by sublaminar wiring. Inspired by this, Ni [4, 5] designed the C1 laminar hook after thorough investigation of atlantoaxial joint anatomy and biomechanics. Combined with C1–C2 transarticular screws and a structural allograft, this technique avoids the risk of spinal cord injury from sublaminar wiring and is easy to manipulate. A biomechanical study confirmed that the bilateral laminar hooks stabilize the allograft and provide equivalent biomechanical stability to bilateral C1–C2 transarticular screw fixation [5]. Clinical evidence shows satisfactory fusion rates and outcomes [4, 6–8].

However, this technique still suffers from drawbacks [9]. It is difficult to connect the hook with the C1–C2 transarticular screws or C2 pedicle screws. The connecting point of the C1 laminar hook is located between the posterior tubercle of the atlas and atlantal lateral mass. This point is more medial compared with the location of the C2 pedicle screw or transarticular screw. The connecting procedure takes some time and effort intraoperatively. Additionally, the hook and screw connection is potentially at risk of loosening or slipping. Considering the unique anatomy of the atlas, we modified the integrated C1 laminar hook with a 15° angle between the hook and the rod to better connect the atlas and the C2 screw. Additionally, the rod can be pre-aligned to better match the regional alignment. Thus, the assembly procedure is easier, more reliable, and safe.

References

1. Dickman CA, Crawford NR, Paramore CG. Biomechanical characteristics of C1–2 cable fixations. J Neurosurg. 1996;85:316–22.
2. Melcher RP, Puttlitz CM, Kleinstueck FS, et al. Biomechanical testing of posterior atlantoaxial fixation techniques. Spine. 2002;27:2435–40.
3. Richter M, Schmidt R, Claes L, et al. Posterior atlantoaxial fixation: biomechanical in vitro comparison of six different techniques. Spine. 2002;27:1724–32.
4. Ni B, Guo X, Xie N, et al. Bilateral atlantoaxial transarticular screws and atlas laminar hooks fixation for pediatric atlantoaxial instability. Spine. 2010;35:E1367–72.
5. Guo X, Ni B, Zhao W, et al. Biomechanical assessment of bilateral C1 laminar hook and C1–2 transarticular screws and bone graft for atlantoaxial instability. J Spinal Disord Tech. 2009;22:578–85.

6. Ni B, Zhou F, Xie N, et al. Transarticular screw and c1 hook fixation for os odontoideum with atlantoaxial dislocation. World Neurosurg. 2011;75:540–6.
7. Ni B, Guo X, Xie N, et al. C1–2 transarticular screws combined with C1 laminar hooks fixation: a modified posterior atlantoaxial fixation technique and outcome in 72 patients. Eur Spine J. 2013;22:260–7.
8. Guo X, Ni B, Xie N, et al. Bilateral C1–C2 transarticular screw and C1 laminar hook fixation and bone graft fusion for reducible atlantoaxial dislocation: a seven-year analysis of outcome. PLoS One. 2014;9:e87676.
9. Xu T, Guo Q, Liu Q, et al. Biomechanical evaluation of a novel integrated C1 laminar hook combined with C1–C2 transarticular screws for atlantoaxial fusion: an in vitro human cadaveric study. World Neurosurg. 2016;92:133–9.

Chapter 12
Manufacture of Integrated C1 Laminar Hooks and C1–C2 Transarticular Screws

Tianming Xu

Abstract The C1 laminar hook that is used currently is a poor match for the C1 posterior arch and is difficult to connect directly to the C1–C2 transarticular screw (TAS). Thus, according to atlantoaxial anatomical features, an integrated C1 laminar hook and C1–C2 transarticular screw were designed, which is safer and more convenient for surgery. This chapter describes the manufacture of integrated C1 laminar hooks and C1–C2 transarticular screws.

12.1 Background of the Design

The anatomical characteristics of the atlantoaxial joint complex include the absence of intervertebral discs, the absence of ligamenta flava, and the distinct shape of C1 and C2. The highly specialized anatomy of this region is designed to provide seemingly paradoxical attributes: loose enough to allow axial rotation and sufficiently tight to protect the delicate structures of the spinal cord and vertebral arteries. The atlantoaxial complex comprises two facet joints and the unique atlantodental articulation. Rotation in the atlantoaxial complex represents 50% of the entire cervical spine rotation.

Trauma, tumor, deformity, and inflammation of the upper cervical spine can cause atlantoaxial instability, and atlantoaxial fixation should be performed for the affected region. Previously, wiring techniques and laminar clamps were used mainly for fixation, the main wiring methods being the Brooks and Gallie techniques [1, 2]. Halifax clamps were also used for single-point fixation [3]. Currently, C1–C2 transarticular screws or short-segment screw fixation is used mainly in atlantoaxial posterior stabilization surgery. Previous biomechanical tests and clinical research have demonstrated that these fixation techniques can enhance the stability of atlantoaxial articulation and improve bone graft fusion [4–10]. It is acknowledged universally that bilateral transarticular screws combined with posterior wiring fixation and bone grafts are the gold standard of atlantoaxial fixation [7, 11–13].

T. Xu
Department of Orthopedics, No. 455 Hospital of PLA, Shanghai, China
e-mail: xutm_smmu@126.com

B. Ni et al. (eds.), *Atlantoaxial Fixation Techniques*, Translational Medicine Research, https://doi.org/10.1007/978-981-10-7889-7_12

Although bilateral C1–C2 transarticular screw (TAS) combined with posterior wiring/cable technique greatly promotes the bone fusion rate of the atlantoaxial complex, it has the risk of spinal cord injury associated with passing the wire/cable sublaminarly. Therefore, bilateral C1 laminar hooks have been used to replace the wire or cable in some studies [14–17]. A new fixation technique for C1–C2 arthrodesis was presented by Ni et al. [18]. It consists of a C1 laminar hook combined with C1–C2 transarticular screws to form an instrument that combines anterior and posterior fixation in the same construct [18]. This bilateral atlantoaxial transarticular screws and atlas laminar hook technique has the advantage over the bilateral transarticular screws combined with posterior wiring fixation because it avoids passing sublaminar wire under the C1 arch. Furthermore, a bone graft can be compressed tightly between the posterior arch of C1 and the lamina of C2 by a rod between the hook and the screw [18]. TAS combined with bilateral C1 laminar hooks represents a three-point fixation, the biomechanical stability of which is comparable to C1–C2 TASs combined with posterior wiring/cable technique [15–18]. However, in clinical practice, we found that the currently used C1 laminar hook is a poor match for the C1 posterior arch and is difficult to connect directly to the C1–C2 TAS. Therefore, according to the atlantoaxial anatomical features, an integrated C1 laminar hook and C1–C2 transarticular screw were designed, which is safer and more convenient for surgery.

12.2 The Theory of the Improvement

For the previous C1 laminar hook, the rods fastened between the hooks and the C1–C2 TAS were complicated, and the assembly was difficult. The poor fit of the C1 laminar hook with the C1 posterior arch poor resulted in unhooking problems. Based on measurements of the C1 posterior arch on human cadaveric cervical spine specimens and CT imaging, a novel integrated C1 laminar hook was designed. It matched the atlantoaxial anatomy well and helped to connect the C1–C2 TAS. Additionally, the design made the hook's contact point on C1 more medial than the current C1 laminar hook, possibly improving its leverage and ability to sandwich a piece of bone effectively.

12.3 Design of the Posterior Integrated C1 Laminar Hook Internal Fixation System

12.3.1 Design Software and Material

The design software used was CAX'A electronic drawing board system from Beijing Beihang Hai'er Software Co., Ltd. (provided by Shanghai Sanyou Medical Instrument Co. Ltd.). The product is made from a titanium alloy that is used frequently for the internal fixation of the spine (Ti6Al4V). This material has higher

Table 12.1 Physical parameters of the titanium alloy

Tensile strength (MPa)	Yield strength (MPa)	Fatigue strength (MPa)	Impact toughness (kg m/cm^2)	Brinell hardness (HB)	Modulus of elasticity (kMPa)	Specific elongation (%)
1055	995	450	3.1	324	110	7.5

fatigue strength than pure implanted titanium, which can prevent hook fracture. Compared with human bones, this material has the best flexibility and rigidity. Its rigidity is 60% that of stainless steel. Its specific gravity is in the range of 4.5–19.3 g/cm^3, which is close to that of human bone. Meanwhile, it has good biochemical and biomechanical compatibility. First, it lacks cytotoxicity, carcinogenicity, teratogenicity, tissue irritation, and immunoreactions. Second, it shows good corrosion resistance, mechanical properties, corrosion fatigue properties, abrasion resistance, and lubrication. Third, it is nonmagnetic, meaning that it will not influence postoperative MRI observations (Table 12.1).

12.3.2 The Shape and Specification of the Posterior Integrated C1 Laminar Hook Internal Fixation System

This internal fixation system consists of screws and integrated C1 laminar hook. After numerous drawing designs, trial manufacture, sample trials, and modifications, the design was finalized.

1. Integrated C1 Laminar Hook and Screw

This novel product integrates a C1 laminar hook and a rod. The main feature was that the rod deviates for 15° outward at the connection with the hook. Furthermore, the rod could be curved to facilitate the connection with the C1–C2 TAS or C2 pedicle screw. Additionally, the integrated design avoids the procedure of connecting a rod to a nonintegrated laminar hook, making the operation more convenient (Figs. 12.1, 12.2, and 12.3).

The atlantoaxial transarticular screw consists of screw body, screw head, and nut. The head of the screw is hollow. The top of the head inclines. It has around 50° incisura. The head of screw has a hole in the center. The body of screw is installed inside. U-shaped grooves are set on both sides of the screw head. The width of the U-shaped grooves matches the outer diameter of the connection rod of the integrated C1 laminar hook. The internal thread is set in the inner wall of the screw head. This internal thread matches the external thread of the nut. The nut is hollow, and the cross section of the cavity is hexagonal, which can be screwed inside the head of screw with matched internal hexagonal wrench. The top of the screw head is inclined 50° incisura; therefore, the body of the screw has a larger range of activity in the incisura surface compared with the head of screw, which meets the requirement of a larger screw angle and screw head angulation in the transarticular space.

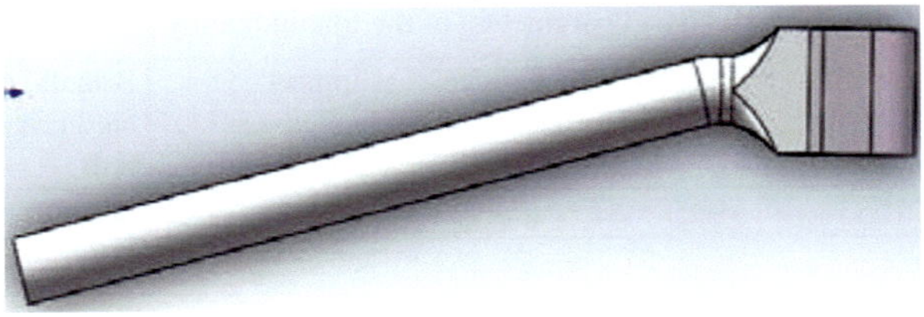

Fig. 12.1 Frontal picture of integrated C1 laminar hook

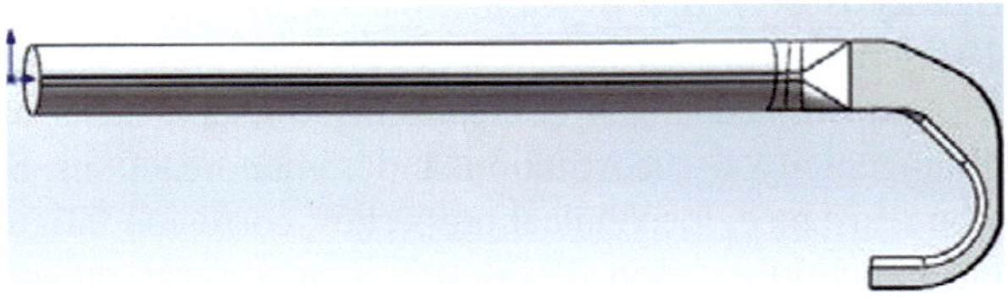

Fig. 12.2 Lateral picture of integrated C1 laminar hook

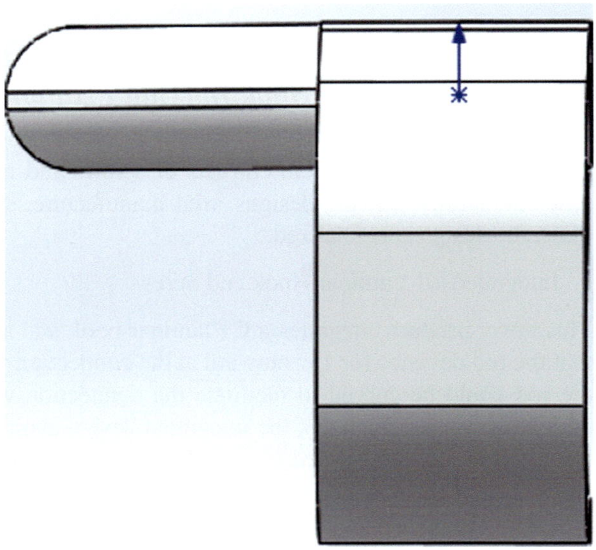

Fig. 12.3 Axial picture of integrated C1 laminar hook

2. Specification

The integrated C1 laminar hook is 4.5 mm wide, the thickness of the body is 3 mm, and the turn of the bilge is 2 mm to the hook tip, which changes gradually to 1.5 mm. The inner diameter varies, for example, it can be 2.8 or 3.0 mm. The length of the rod is 40 mm, and the outer diameter is 3 mm. The outer diameter of the multiaxial screw body can be 3.5 or 4.0 mm, and the length can range from 24 to 44 mm, in increments of 2 mm. The inner diameter of the head of screw matches that of the outer diameter of the nut (7.8 mm).

12.3.3 Manufacturing Process

The main manufacturing processes are mechanical processing, bending, grinding, abrasive blasting, oxidization, lettering, washing, and packaging. Mechanical processing can be performed in several ways. For the best precision, we used turn-mill combination primary processing. The processing tool was a Swiss turn-milling combined machine, whose tool number was WM-508MT. The material used was a 25-mm titanium alloy rod. The rod end was processed to the size required, and milling processing is conducted for the hook part. Finally, a self-centering vice clamp was used to control the components. Milling tool was used to cut off the components. After turning over by the vice to mill the remaining part, the components are fed into the work bin of the machine tool automatically. Bending is completed by a bench worker according to the angles required in the drawings. First, a mold was made that fits the bended shape, and the components are placed into the mold to be bent and shaped on the press machine. Grinding was used mainly to remove the fine lines from the surface. The magnetic grinding miller used vibrating friction with a stainless steel pin to make the surface of component bright. Ceramic beads (200-mesh) can be used for the abrasive blasting process. After abrasive blasting of the surface of the components, a matte effect was achieved. After abrasive blasting, it can be oxidized into different colors according to various specifications. After oxidization, characters can be carved by a laser on the surface of a component. After which the products are washed, packaged, and stored.

Product inspection comprised measuring the dimensional tolerance marked on the drawings. No scars on the surface resulting from processing and bending are permitted, and the surface should be smooth and even. A component that did not meet the requirement of the tolerance range was scrapped. A component that has defects on its surface was examined as to whether it should be reprocessed or scrapped according to the actual situation. The color after oxidization, which should be uniform without fire burn, was compared with the color card.

12.4 Design and Functional Characteristics

The size of integrated C1 laminar hook is chosen according to the human cervical vertebra anatomy. The hook should be able to be placed into the arcus posterior atlantis and controlled stably. In addition, the volume should be minimized to prevent stimulating the surrounding tissues. The rod end of the integrated C1 laminar hook will match the screw (diameter 3.5 mm). The length of rod end is also obtained according to the anatomical data and divided into X specifications. The width of the screw seat of the C1–C2 transarticular screw or C2 pedicle screw should exceed the width of the installation site of the integrated hook. For the convenience of installing the hook onto the seat of the C2 screw, a dip angle should be set between the rod end and the hook. According to analysis of the anatomical data, this angle should be 15°.

1. The integrated design of the C1 laminar hook and rod reduces assembly links during surgery and is convenient for connection. In addition, the hook can adhere better to the arcus posterior atlantis, which increases the contact surface and decreases concentration of stress. Different sized hooks are available for the people with different posterior arches of the atlas, and it is not necessary to bite the bone substance to fit the size of the hook.
2. A protuberant ridge was designed into the contact area between the hook and the C1 posterior arch, which reduces sliding of the hook on the C1 posterior arch, making it difficult to move.
3. The unique extroversion design makes it possible to connect the C1–C2 transarticular screws or C2 pedicles to vertebral arch directly. While jointly entrapping the bone grafts, it can also limit bone graft shift, which is an advantage.
4. The head of the atlantoaxial multiaxial screw inclined at around 50° incisura. Thus, the body of screw has a large range of activity on the incisura surface compared with the screw head, which meets the requirement of a larger screw angle and screw head angulation in the transarticular space, making it convenient to connect the screw head and the connecting rod, and it reduces the stress concentration in the joint between the screw head and the screw body.
5. The atlas laminar hook can lock the bone grafting block to avoid coming off and increase the stability.

12.5 Installation of the Posterior Integrated Hook Atlantoaxial Internal Fixation System

The operation should be conducted under C-shaped x-ray machine imaging. The inlet of the screw is in the sagittal line through the isthmus ridge of the inferior margin of the C2 vertebral plate. At 20 mm from where the inner margin of the C2 zygopophysis projects upward and outward, a hand drill is used to open a cortical bone window in the inlet; the drill is also used to drill into the C2 pedicle of vertebral arch carefully, and the most suitable direction is decided according to perspective conditions. The drill works forward along the sagittal plane, adjoining the facies medialis of the isthmus of the C2 pedicle of the vertebral arch across the posterior of that atlantoaxial joint to enter the lateral mass of the atlas. To prevent breaking the cortex of the bone, or damaging the vertebral artery and intraspinal spinal cord, a round-head probe is used to detect the depth of the screw path and peripheral wall to make sure the bone tunnel is not broken through. The suitable length of screw is selected. After screw tap is used to tap screw path, the multiaxial cortical bone screw can be screwed carefully along the screw path. After the operation is completed, the same technique can be used to imbed the opposite screw, and the head of screw can be 50° upward from the incisura to keep the head of the screw at the same level. Afterward, the hook of the integrated C1 laminar hook is hung carefully over the posterior arch of the atlas along the inside wall of posterior arch. The connecting rod is put into the

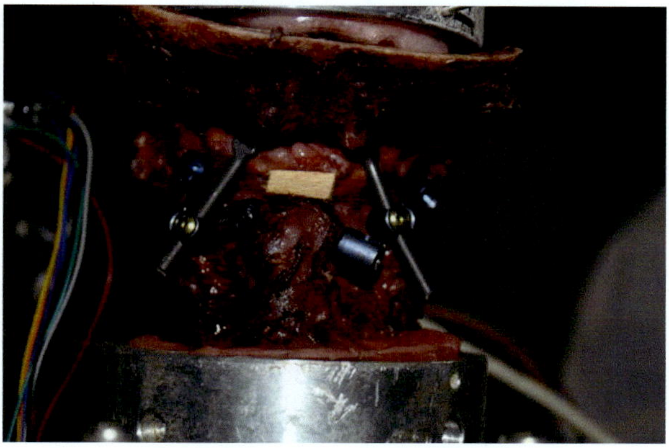

Fig. 12.4 A specimen fixed with integrated C1 laminar hooks

U-shaped groove of the head of the C1–C2 transarticular screw, screwing in the nut as a temporary fixation. The T-shaped spongy bone that has a double-clear bone cortex is incised from the right posterior superior iliac spine. The bone grafting bed is cleaned, and a high-speed drill is used to grind the cortex of bone on the surface of the posterior arch of the atlas and the cortex of the bone on the superior border of the axial vertebral plate. The assembled and shaped ilium graft is impacted between the posterior arch of the atlas and the C2 spinous process, imbedded into the integrated connecting rod. A pressing clamp is used to press the bilateral inner fixed system, clamping the bone grafting block between posterior arch of the atlas and the C2 spinous process. Meanwhile, the atlas laminar hook is better adhered and imbedded into the posterior arch of the atlas by locking the nut of the transarticular screw. Therefore, bone grafting pressing fixation of the unstable atlas-axis is completed via an integrated laminar hook and C1–C2 transarticular screw to fix the posterior arch of the atlas, the bone grafting block, and the C2 vertebral plate (Fig. 12.4).

References

1. Harms J, Melcher RP. Posterior C1–C2 fusion with polyaxial screw and rod fixation. Spine. 2001;15:2467–71.
2. Dickman CA, Crawford NR, Paramore CG. Biomechanical characteristics of C1–C2 cable fixations. J Neurosurg. 1996;85:316–22.
3. Dickman CA, Sonnag VK. Posterior C1–C2 transarticular screw fixation for atlantoaxial arthrodesis. J Neurosurg. 1998;43:275–80.
4. Grob D, Crisco JJ, Panjabi MM, et al. Biomechanical evaluation of four different posterior atlantoaxial fixation techniques. Spine. 1992;17:480–90.
5. Hanson PB, Montesano PX, Sharkey NA, et al. Anatomic and biomechanical assessment of transarticular screw fixation for atlantoaxial instability. Spine. 1991;16:1141–5.
6. Montesano PX, Juach EC, Anderson PA, et al. Biomechanics of cervical spine internal fixation. Spine. 1991;16(Suppl 3):S10–6.

7. Naderi S, Crawford NR, Song GS, et al. Biomechanical comparison of C1–C2 posterior fixations. Cable, graft, and screw combinations. Spine. 1998;23:1946–55.
8. Smith MD, Kotzar G, Yoo J, et al. A biomechanical analysis of atlantoaxial stabilization methods using a bovine model: C1–C2 fixation analysis. Clin Orthop. 1993;290:285–95.
9. Wilke H-J, Fischer K, Kugler A, et al. In vitro investigations of internal fixation systems of the upper cervical spine: II. Stability of posterior atlantoaxial fixation techniques. Eur Spine J. 1992;1:191–9.
10. Melcher RP, Puttlitz CM, Kleinstueck FS, et al. Biomechanical testing of posterior atlantoaxial fixation techniques. Spine. 2002;27:2435–40.
11. Richter M, Schmidt R, Claes L, et al. Posterior atlantoaxial fixation: biomechanical in vitro comparison of six different techniques. Spine. 2002;27:1724–32.
12. Elgafy H, Potluri T, Goel VK, et al. Biomechanical analysis comparing three C1–C2 transarticular screw salvaging fixation techniques. Spine. 2010;35:378–85.
13. Sim HB, Lee JW, Park JT, et al. Biomechanical evaluations of various c1–c2 posterior fixation techniques. Spine. 2011;36:E401–7.
14. Guo X, Ni B, Xie N, Lu X, Guo Q, Lu M. Bilateral C1–C2 transarticular screw and C1 laminar hook fixation and bone graft fusion for reducible atlantoaxial dislocation: a seven-year analysis of outcome. PLoS One. 2014;9(1):e87676.
15. Ni B, Guo X, Xie N, Li S, Zhou F, Zhang F, et al. C1–2 transarticular screws combined with C1 laminar hooks fixation: a modified posterior atlantoaxial fixation technique and outcome in 72 patients. Eur Spine J. 2013;22(2):260–7.
16. Guo X, Ni B, Wang M, Wang J, Li S, Zhou F. Bilateral atlas laminar hook combined with transarticular screw fixation for an unstable bursting atlantal fracture. Arch Orthop Trauma Surg. 2009;129(9):1203–9.
17. Ni B, Zhou F, Xie N, Guo X, Yang L, Guo Q, et al. Transarticular screw and c1 hook fixation for os odontoideum with atlantoaxial dislocation. World Neurosurg. 2011;75(3–4):540–6.
18. Guo X, Ni B, Zhao W, et al. Biomechanical assessment of bilateral C1 laminar hook and C1–2 transarticular screws and bone graft for atlantoaxial instability. J Spinal Disord Tech. 2009;22:578–85.

Chapter 13
Introduction of a Novel Integrated C1 Laminar Hook Combined with C1–C2 Transarticular Screws for Atlantoaxial Fixation

Qi Liu and Tianming Xu

Abstract In practice, C1–C2 transarticular screw (TAS) combined with bilateral C1 laminar hooks could be used for atlantoaxial instability to avoid the risk of spinal cord injury which is usually caused by sublaminar wire inserting. But, a standard C1 laminar hook does not match the posterior arch of C1 well, and to connect it with the C1–C2 TAS is difficult. To solve this problem, we have designed an integrated C1 laminar hook based on measurement data acquired from human cadaveric cervical spine specimens and computed tomography images. This hook matches the atlanto-axial anatomy perfectly and facilitates connection to the C1–C2 TAS. Furthermore, the more medial contact point of this hook on C1 potentially improves leverage and the ability to clamp a block of bone graft tight. The biomechanical characteristics of this new C1 hook have been tested on human cadaveric specimens and compared with other internal fixation techniques commonly used [1].

In practice, C1–C2 transarticular screw (TAS) combined with bilateral C1 laminar hooks could be used for atlantoaxial instability to avoid the risk of spinal cord injury which is usually caused by sublaminar wire inserting. But, a standard C1 laminar hook does not match the posterior arch of C1 well, and to connect it with the C1–C2 TAS is difficult. To solve this problem, we have designed an integrated C1 laminar hook based on measurement data acquired from human cadaveric cervical spine specimens and computed tomography images. This hook matches the atlantoaxial anatomy perfectly and facilitates connection to the C1–C2 TAS. Furthermore, the more medial contact point of this hook on C1 potentially improves leverage and the ability to clamp a block of bone graft tight. The biomechanical characteristics of this

Q. Liu (✉)
Department of Orthopedics, The First Affiliated Hospital of Xiamen University, Xiamen, China

T. Xu
Department of Orthopedics, No. 455 Hospital of PLA, Shanghai, China

B. Ni et al. (eds.), *Atlantoaxial Fixation Techniques*, Translational Medicine Research, https://doi.org/10.1007/978-981-10-7889-7_13

new C1 hook have been tested on human cadaveric specimens and compared with other internal fixation techniques commonly used [1].

In our study, seven human cervical spine specimens (Oc-C3) were involved. The specimens were tested on the MTS 858 Mini Bionix II test system in six directions under torque control mode (1.5 nm), and the motions were captured by an optoelectronic motion analysis system. Each specimen was tested under four conditions: (1) intact, (2) destabilized (type II odontoid fracture mode), and (3) different internal fixations after destabilized, including (a) bilateral C1–C2 TAS combined with wire and bone graft (TAS+G), (b) bilateral C1–C2 TAS combined with the new C1 laminar hook (TAS+H), (c) C1 lateral mass screw and C2 pedicle screw (C2PS+C1LMS), and (d) the integrated C1 laminar hooks combined with C2 pedicle screws (C2PS+H).

The mean C1–C2 ROM of the intact group was 63.43° ± 3.22° in axial rotation, 22.60° ± 4.93° in flexion/extension, and 11.40° ± 2.58° in lateral bending. The mean ROM for the destabilization group was significantly increased in all directions relative to that for the intact group. As we can imagine, the C1–C2 ROMs for all the fixation groups in all directions were significantly decreased compared with those for the intact group and destabilization group.

Among the fixation groups, the greatest mean C1–C2 ROM during axial rotation was found in the C2PS+H group. However, there was no significant difference between the C2PS+H and the other three fixation groups during flexion/extension or lateral bending (all $P > 0.05$). The details of this study can be seen in our published article [1].

Hence, we can conclude that the TAS+H technique can achieve instant stability comparable to that achieved with the TAS+G technique for treating C1–C2 instability. The C2PS+H technique is a reliable alternative biomechanically, despite the less stability during axial rotation than the other three techniques.

Reference

1. Xu T, Guo Q, Liu Q, Zhang P, Lu M, Lu X, Chen F, Guo X, Ni B. Biomechanical evaluation of a novel integrated C1 laminar hook combined with C1–C2 transarticular screws for atlantoaxial fusion: an in vitro human cadaveric study. World Neurosurg. 2016;92:133–9. https://doi.org/10.1016/j.wneu.2016.04.126.

Chapter 14
Atlas Lateral Mass Long-Tail Reduction Screw: Axis Pedicle Screw and Rod Fixation Technique

Jun Yang

Abstract This chapter describes the reduction technique for atlantoaxial dislocation using C1 long-tail reduction lateral mass screw and C2 pedicle screw. Firstly, the spondylolisthesis long-tail reduction screws at the atlas and pedicle screws of the axis are placed, and the rods to the screws of the axis are locked. Then, the nuts of C1 long-tail reduction lateral mass screw are gradually fastened. As a result, the screw-rod lever system distracts the atlas backward and pushes the axis downward and forward, thus achieving reduction of the atlantoaxial joint dislocation.

Instability of the atlantoaxial joint may be a result of congenital anomalies, degeneration, infectious diseases, injury or trauma, disorders, and/or surgery. Therefore, the use of atlantoaxial fusion and stabilization procedures to restore atlantoaxial stability is increasing.

Surgical strategies have evolved over time. Initially, atlantoaxial instability typically was treated using a variety of wiring constructs, such as the Brooks or Gallie techniques. However, these techniques depend on an intact posterior arch of C1. Any sublaminar wiring technique (typically under the C1 ring and/or under the C2 lamina) requires adequate room in the spinal canal to avoid neurological injury. This is most often an issue with a fixed C1 on C2 subluxation in a rheumatoid arthritis patient, where the cord space at the C1 level can be severely compromised. In addition, wiring techniques are less biomechanically favorable than screw fixation in terms of rotation and lateral bending; thus, they often require halo stabilization [1–3]. In 1987, atlantoaxial arthrodesis using transarticular screws was first described by Magerl and Seeman [4]. The major advantage of atlantoaxial transarticular screw fixation is the provision of rigid fixation. This technique gets good fusion rate and no need of postoperative halo immobilization in most cases. It also allows for atlantoaxial fusion in cases without an intact posterior arch of the atlas. However, this technique requires reduction of the atlantoaxial joint complex before placement of instrumentation.

J. Yang
Department of Orthopedics, Changzheng Hospital, Shanghai, China
e-mail: yangjunspine@hotmail.com

B. Ni et al. (eds.), *Atlantoaxial Fixation Techniques*, Translational Medicine Research, https://doi.org/10.1007/978-981-10-7889-7_14

In 1994, Goel firstly described a screw-plate fixation technique of the atlas and the axis; the screws were placed into the lateral mass of the atlas and the C2 pedicle [5]. Jürgen Harms modified this technique, who developed a screw-rod fixation technique. The technique is more adaptable for use with polyaxial screw-rod system, which will preserve the nerve root of C2, and easy to operate in fractures and dislocations of the atlas [6]. With a full understanding of anatomical and biomechanical studies, other authors suggested that screws should be placed directly through the posterior arch of C1, just above Harms' technique entry point [7, 8]. This technique also can avoid venous plexus hemorrhage and damage to the C2 root. This technique also theoretically improves the pullout strength of the C1 screw by increasing the length of screw fixation within the bone. However, morphometric studies have shown that this technique is limited by the size of the posterior arch and is not always feasible. In 709 atlas specimens measured bilaterally, Lee [9] et al. found that only 46.2% had a posterior arch thickness greater than 4 mm and only 13.7% were greater than 5 mm. Tan et al. [10] found that only 4 of the 50 C1 specimens (8%) had a posterior arch thickness less than 4 mm. They also reported that ten C1 lateral mass screws were successfully placed in five patients using this technique.

Our reduction screw technique is different from the techniques mentioned above and is modified from Harms' technique. Most atlantoaxial joint dislocation cases are anterolisthesis of the atlas over the axis, similar to lumbar spondylolisthesis. Therefore, this problem can be addressed by placing spondylolisthesis long-tail reduction screws at the atlas and by locking the rods to the screws of the axis first and then gradually fastening them with locking nuts; the screw-rod lever system distracts the atlas backward and pushes the axis downward and forward, thus achieving reduction of the atlantoaxial joint dislocation. In our series cases, we used C1 long-tail reduction lateral mass screw–C2 pedicle screw and rod fixation system for surgery of the upper cervical spine. In the technique, the screws are placed through the arch into the lateral mass of C1. Combined with our clinical practice, we find that drilling through the posterior arch of atlas will be difficult and can injure the vertebral artery (VA) or C2 root bundle if the arch is less than 5 mm wide. In this technique, it was easy to put the rods into the tails of the atlas screws. By contrast, extra reduction forceps are no longer needed to perform the reduction of the atlas in the limited operative space. This reduction screw technique can achieve immediate fixation after reduction, with advantages of procedural simplicity and good results. Our choice of the common indications includes type II odontoid fractures, atlantoaxial instability in patients with rheumatoid arthritis, and iatrogenic instability after anterior odontoid resection for the treatment of basilar invagination. Other causes of atlantoaxial instability, such as Down syndrome, may also be treated using this technique. This technique also can be used for more flexibility in cases of aberrant VA or cases with destruction of the C1–C2 joint result from bony abnormalities. The fusion rate of the associated fixation method exceeds 90% [11–13]. There are two significant advantages compared to Magerl's technique. Firstly, C2 pedicle screw is much easier to place with no much demanded angle. Secondly, it is very useful for treating the cases of a dislocated or fractured atlas.

During surgery, the lateral mass of C1 is identified using blunt dissection, just inferior to the C1 ring, and approximately 2–3 cm lateral to the midline. We used to choose the entry point in the middle of the posterior lateral mass and at the top of the arcuate surface. A 2 mm burr is used to score the starting point. A hand drill is then used to insert a drill bit to a depth of approximately 1 cm, and the trajectory is confirmed using anteroposterior (AP) and lateral fluoroscopic visualization. The trajectory for screw placement is slightly medialized (5–10°) and is parallel to the posterior arch in the sagittal plane. When placing C2 pedicle screws, the entry point is usually 3 mm above the C2–C3 joint and more farther lateral than that for the transarticular or C2 par screws. In practice, placing C2 pedicle screws is no much better than placing C2 par screws, but the associated VA injury risk is higher [13]. C2 laminar screws are another alternative screw fixations, which required an intact C2 lamina (Figs. 14.1, 14.2, 14.3, and 14.4).

Next, the C2 screws are locked and the rods are contoured to the approximate cervical lordosis before placing. For larger slips, C1 was instrumented with long-tail reduction lateral mass screws. Figure 14.2 shows the placement of screws with the posterior rod contoured in approximation of the cervical lordosis before reduction. By gradually fastening the locking nuts of the C1 screws, the screw-rod lever system displaces the atlas backward and pushes the axis downward and forward, so C1 screw is slowly pulled back until to the same level of the C2 screws. Intermittent distraction is very important for the maneuver to achieve good reduction of the displacement.

After removing the cortical bone of the caudal edge of the C1 posterior arch and the cranial edge of the C2 laminar and spinous process, an autologous iliac bone graft is harvested and modified according to the bilateral shape. The height of the bone graft will be bigger than the interval distance of C1 posterior arch and C2 lamina, and then the graft is pushed between C1 and C2. Use tools to verify the tight of the graft in place after longitudinal pressure on both C1 and C2 screw sides.

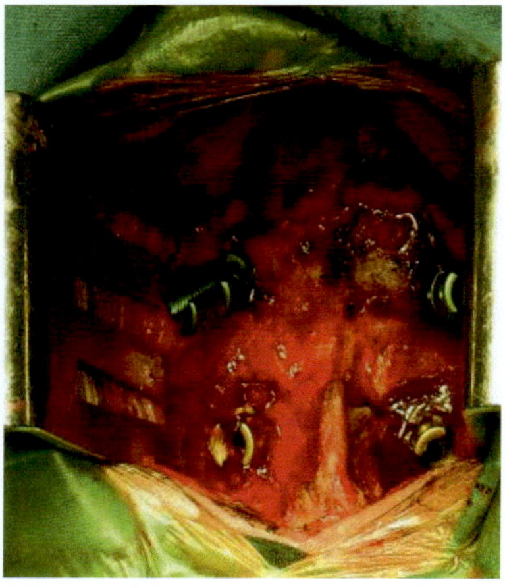

Fig. 14.1 Intraoperative placement of bilateral atlas long-tail drawing back reduction pedicle screws and axis pedicle screws

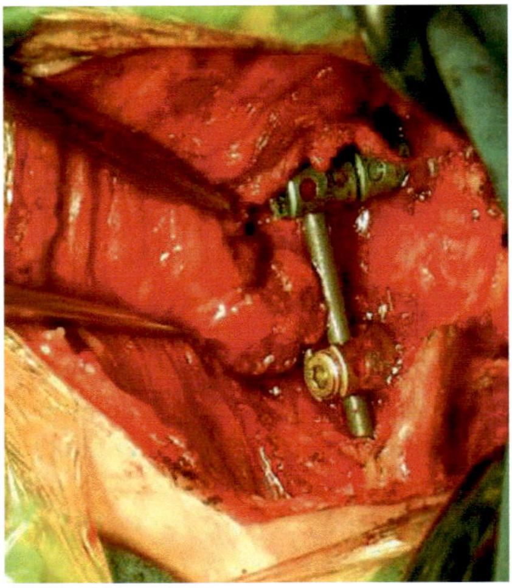

Fig. 14.2 Adjustment of the connecting rod for pulling reduction

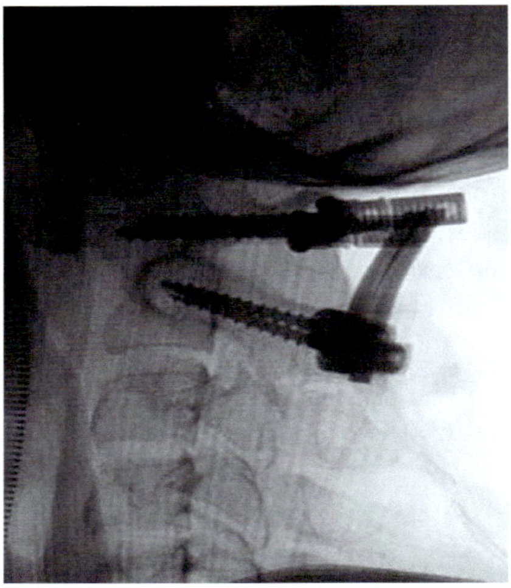

Fig. 14.3 Perspective view after adjustment of the connecting rod

Our study shows that the reduction screw technique has achieved good long-lasting stability. Several biomechanical studies have also been performed to assess the pullout strength of C1 and C2 fixation screws that were placed using various techniques. Hong et al. [14] showed almost equivalent pullout strengths between C1 lateral mass screws (1716.16 N) and C2 pedicle screws (1631.94 N). Similarly, Hott et al. [15] demonstrated a mean pullout strength of 667 N using bicortical C1 lateral mass fixation, which was comparable to the pullout strength of C2 pars screws (556 N). In 2007, Eck et al. [16] reported a statistically significant ($P = 0.006$) increase in the pullout strength of C1 lateral mass screws placed with bicortical versus unicortical purchase. They questioned the necessity of using bicortical fixation routinely, given the greater pullout strength of unicortical C1 lateral mass screws when compared with that of subaxial lateral mass screws reported in other studies.

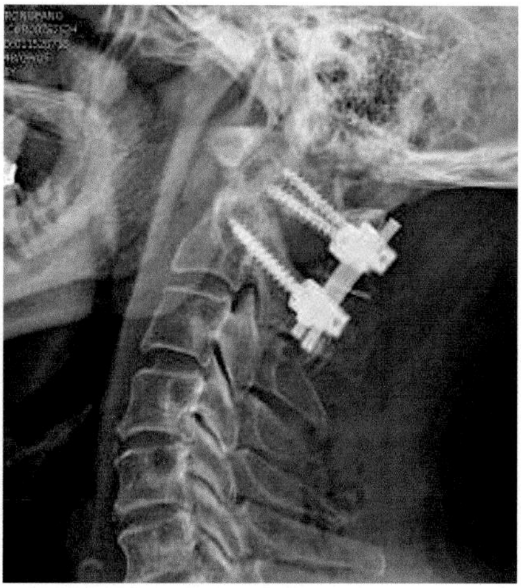

Fig. 14.4 Postoperative lateral roentgenographs showing the good position of screw fixation and reduction of the atlas

They also noted the increased risk of injury to structures anterior to the C1 lateral mass that can occur with bicortical screw placement. In 2009, Ma [17] compared the pullout strength of C1 lateral mass screws (placed in the lateral mass with Harms' technique) versus the pedicle screws (placed through the posterior arch to the lateral mass) and with unicortical versus bicortical purchase. Unicortical lateral mass screws provided the weakest fixation (mean, 794.5 N) and bicortical pedicle screws the strongest (1757.0 N). However, there were no statistically significant differences between bicortical C1 lateral mass screws (1243.8 N) and unicortical C1 pedicle screws (1192.5 N). Furthermore, there was also no statistically significant difference in biomechanical construct stability between bicortical C1 lateral mass screw-rod constructs and unicortical C1 pedicle screw-rod constructs. Thus, in our cases, we place unicortical pedicle screws in C1 as an alternative to placing bicortical C1 lateral mass screws.

Our long-tail reduction screw technique via a C1 long-tail reduction lateral mass screw–C2 pedicle screw and rod fixation system, followed by an autologous iliac bone graft fusion, is a safe and effective procedure for atlantoaxial joint dislocation.

References

1. Dickman CA, Sonntag VKH, Papadopoulos SM, Hadley MN. The interspinous method of posterior atlantoaxial arthrodesis. J Neurosurg. 1991;74(2):190–8.
2. Grob D, Crisco JJ III, Panjabi MM, Wang P, Dvorak J. Biomechanical evaluation of four different posterior atlantoaxial fixation techniques. Spine. 1992;17(5):480–90.
3. Hanley EN Jr, Harvell JC Jr. Immediate postoperative stability of the atlantoaxial articulation: a biomechanical study comparing simple midline wiring, and the Gallie and Brooks procedures. J Spinal Disord. 1992;5(3):306–10.

4. Magerl F, Seemann PS. Stable posterior fusion of the atlas and axis by transarticular screw fixation. In: Kehr P, Weidner A, editors. Cervical spine I. New York: Springer; 1987. p. 322–7.
5. Goel A, Laheri V. Plate and screw fixation for atlanto-axial subluxation. Acta Neurochir. 1994; 129(1–2):47–53.
6. Harms J, Melcher RP. Posterior C1–C2 fusion with polyaxial screw and rod fixation. Spine. 2001;26(22):2467–71.
7. MacKenzie AI, Uttley D, Marsh HT, Bell BA. Craniocervical stabilization using Luque/Hartshill rectangles. Neurosurgery. 1990;26(1):32–6.
8. Resnick DK, Lapsiwala S, Trost GR. Anatomic suitability of the C1–C2 complex for pedicle screw fixation. Spine. 2002;27(14):1494–8.
9. Lee MJ, Cassinelli E, Riew KD. The feasibility of inserting atlas lateral mass screws via the posterior arch. Spine. 2006;31(24):2798–801.
10. Tan M, Wang H, Wang Y, et al. Morphometric evaluation of screw fixation in atlas via posterior arch and lateral mass. Spine. 2003;28(9):888–95.
11. Parker SL, McGirt MJ, Garcés-Ambrossi GL, et al. Translaminar versus pedicle screw fixation of C2: comparison of surgical morbidity and accuracy of 313 consecutive screws. Neurosurgery. 2009;64(5, Suppl 2):343–8.
12. Acosta FL Jr, Quinones-Hinojosa A, Gadkary CA, et al. Frameless stereotactic image-guided C1–C2 transarticular screw fixation for atlantoaxial instability: review of 20 patients. J Spinal Disord Tech. 2005;18(5):385–91.
13. Mummaneni PV, Lu DC, Dhall SS, Mummaneni VP, Chou D. C1 lateral mass fixation: a comparison of constructs. Neurosurgery. 2010;66(3, Suppl):153–60.
14. Hong X, Dong Y, Yunbing C, Qingshui Y, Shizheng Z, Jingfa L. Posterior screw placement on the lateral mass of atlas: an anatomic study. Spine. 2004;29(5):500–3.
15. Hott JS, Lynch JJ, Chamberlain RH, et al. Biomechanical comparison of C1–2 posterior fixation techniques. J Neurosurg Spine. 2005;2(2):175–81.
16. Eck JC, Walker MP, Currier BL, et al. Biomechanical comparison of unicortical versus bicortical C1 lateral mass screw fixation. J Spinal Disord Tech. 2007;20(7):505–8.
17. Ma XY, Yin QS, Wu ZH, et al. C1 pedicle screws versus C1 lateral mass screws: comparisons of pullout strengths and biomechanical stabilities. Spine. 2009;34(4):371–7.

Part IV

Design, Development, and Marketing of an Integrated Screw-Hook System for Posterior Atlas-Axis Fixation

Abstract

Traditionally, hospitals and doctors passively receive medical devices from manufacturers. In this research project, hospitals and doctors had closer relationships with the manufacturers to co-develop a new integrated cervical screw-hook system. Changzheng Hospital provided doctors' ideas derived from fundamental research data, while Shanghai Sanyou Medical Co., Ltd. provided efficient and precise designs and experimental platforms. The product underwent several key processes: design verification, cadaver operation, finite element analysis, biomechanical tests, standard implant mechanic tests, biocompatibility tests, risk assessments, mass production, and quality control. Market analysis, life cycle analysis, and clinical feedback for the integrated screw-hook system are also discussed.

Chapter 15
Research Collaboration Between Doctors and Manufacturers

Yuli Ma

Abstract Traditionally, manufacturers develop new devices and provide them to hospitals via distributors, and the doctors use the products to cure patients. In the modern information-based society, the development, production, evaluation, and distribution of products are experiencing significant changes. The combination of advantages and integration of superior resources becomes one of the most important methods to develop medical devices. Orthopedic devices are particularly specialized and are usually developed via cooperation between doctors and the device manufacturer. The product can only be developed when all three concerns are satisfied, which are clinical need, technical feasibility, and company interest. The cooperation partner must have professional R&D group and facilities and an advanced quality assurance system.

15.1 Hospital-Institute-Company Cooperation and the Win-Win Mode

Traditionally, manufacturers develop new devices and provide them to hospitals via distributors, and the doctors use the products to cure patients. However, this is only part of the development process. Original ideas for new devices often arise as a result of doctor's clinical practice while treating patients, leading to improvement or innovation of existing therapies. Usually, these thoughts and ideas need to be realized in the form of new devices, which when developed lead to improvements to existing therapies. This generates a corresponding market demand for such improvements. Companies can increase demand by gathering market data, inputting resources, cooperating with doctors to develop products, and utilizing suitable distributors to maximize market penetration. With the increased use of existing products, doctors can make further innovations, thus creating a beneficial cycle for the entire industry.

Y. Ma
Shanghai Sanyou Medical Co. Ltd, Shanghai, China
e-mail: yuli.ma@sanyou-medical.com

B. Ni et al. (eds.), *Atlantoaxial Fixation Techniques*, Translational Medicine Research, https://doi.org/10.1007/978-981-10-7889-7_15

In the modern information-based society, the development, production, evaluation, and distribution of products are experiencing significant changes. For medical devices, massive data mining and accumulation provide a solid basis for treatment; the development of industrial design and 3D printing techniques have shortened the research cycle greatly; and the finite element method (FEM) and biomechanical experiments assure the reliability of new products. These technological innovations have reduced the development time of medical devices significantly. However, the requirements for economical and intelligence resources are even more important. Hence, the combination of advantages and integration of superior resources becomes one of the most important methods to develop medical devices.

Orthopedic devices are particularly specialized and are usually developed via cooperation between doctors and the device manufacturer. With orthopedic devices, doctors have most authority to determine the requirements for the products. In cooperation with engineers, doctors can transfer their ideas into practical designs and, eventually, products. This has become a routine method in the orthopedic industry in recent years.

Unfortunately, not all ideas become products. Product development is usually based on company strategies. Figure 15.1 shows the three main concerns of company strategies: clinical need, technical feasibility, and company interest. The product can only be developed when all three concerns are satisfied. Clinical need include clinical demand, therapeutic innovation, and product regeneration. Technical feasibility includes support from existing materials, techniques, laws and regulations, therapeutic recognition, doctors' surgical skills, and company resources. The company interest usually regard long-term profitability after resource input. The physical development is undertaken by research and development (R&D) programs. R&D programs comprise two parts: research programs and product development pro-

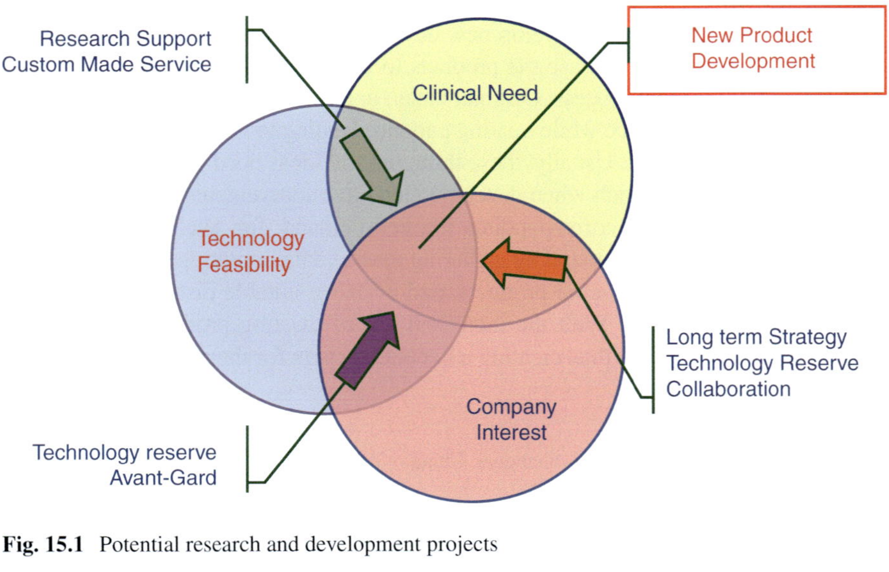

Fig. 15.1 Potential research and development projects

grams. Even when the main concerns are not all satisfied, the company will support research programs to enhance collaboration with doctors, to explore new technical availability, or to increase the R&D ability of the company.

Therefore, for a hospital with a complete research and surgical system in the orthopedic area, it is of utmost importance to find a high-quality device manufacturer to integrate resource advantages and to provide strong R&D support to develop new devices. Thus, hospitals can provide better services to patients by getting timely feedback, turning thoughts into products faster, and making products more reliable. The company can then benefit socially and economically by gathering therapeutic experiences, increasing R&D efficiency, and shortening development time cycles.

During the development of the integrated screw-hook system, we cooperated comprehensively with Shanghai Sanyou Medical Co., Ltd. (be hereafter referred to as Sanyou Medical). During the development period, Sanyou Medical undertook the improvement and manufacture of a prototype of an internal fixation system based on patents provided by the hospital. After FEM and biomechanical experiments, the company made further improvements to the design of the system and manufactured the final products. The hospital provided patents and performed in vitro biomechanical experiments. Both sides shared the patents and profits. By such cooperation, clinical problems were resolved by inventing new devices, which increased their clinical effectiveness and steered doctors toward practical products of high value with both economic and social benefits. The products were manufactured by Chinese local company and were suitable for Chinese patients. The cooperative process also increased the self-development experience of both sides and built a solid foundation for further cooperation.

15.2 The Qualifications and Requirements of a Cooperation Partner

The cooperation partner must have the following qualifications:

1. Professional R&D group and facilities. Compared with other industries, orthopedic device development demands more professional and skilled engineers. The R&D of orthopedic devices is a special interdisciplinary field. R&D engineers must have good understanding of anatomy, pathology, and surgery, as well as a solid knowledge of design, experimentation, and manufacture. The engineers do not take part in the practical treatment or surgery; therefore, their knowledge can only be obtained through cooperation with doctors in long-term programs. Unfortunately, in China, the manufacturer of orthopedic devices is a relatively new industry, and there is a lack of talent. Professional facilities can be divided into three categories: (1) hardware/software systems, numerical anatomy models, material and structural experiment systems, numerical analysis systems, and reference design databases for product design; (2) biomechanical experiment systems, FEM simulation systems, and material/structural characterization systems

used for fundamental research; and (3) hardware/software systems for prototype manufacture and process research. We will use Tytus Laboratories (be hereafter referred to as Tytus Labs) of Sanyou Medical as an example to demonstrate the basic structure and facilities of a professional R&D department (Fig. 15.2).

2. An advanced quality assurance system. Similar to other industries, the production of orthopedic devices must follow strict, reasonable, and reliable quality assurance systems to maintain the effectiveness and safety of the products. We will introduce the quality assurance system and specific research process of Tytus Labs in the following sections.

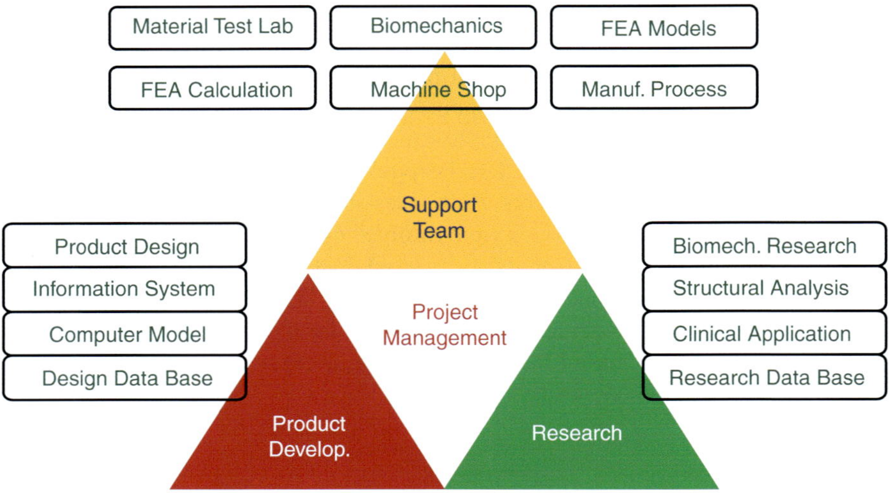

Fig. 15.2 R&D structure (Tytus Labs)

Chapter 16
Integrated Screw-Hook Development

Michael Mingyan Liu

Abstract The development of spinal products must obey strict quality assurance guidelines. The uniqueness of orthopedic R&D is reflected in the requirements of the main steps: product design, strength analysis and structural optimization, functional analysis and evaluation, and surgical evaluation. Design process of the Integrated Screw-Hook System by Sanyou Medical includes design evaluation and validation, cadaver surgery, FEM simulations, biomechanical experiments, mechanical experiments on the implants, biocompatibility test of materials, and risk assessment evaluation of design. Industrial production process and product quality control are also discussed.

16.1 The R&D Process and Quality Assurance System for Orthopedic Products

The development of spinal products must obey strict quality assurance guidelines. The common method for medical device development is based on the design control requirement—21 CFR 820.30, which was established by the Food and Drug Administration (FDA) in 1990 [1]. That document clarifies the requirements of the R&D process, as well as defines and explains the main steps of the process, such as design input, regular evaluation, verification, validation, and transfer. The international standard ISO 13485 [2] also proposes similar suggestions and guidance for the R&D of medical devices such that the quality assurance system satisfies MDD 93/42/EEC [3] published by the European Union. Companies should establish an R&D process that suits the domestic situation by following these guidelines. The following chart (Fig. 16.1) shows the R&D process of Tytus Labs of Sanyou Medical.

The uniqueness of orthopedic R&D is reflected in the requirements of the main steps. Here, we will only discuss about several steps directly related with final products, omitting the details of the other steps, process check points, and details in design history files.

M. M. Liu
Shanghai Sanyou Medical Co. Ltd, Shanghai, China
e-mail: mingyan.liu@sanyou-medical.com

B. Ni et al. (eds.), *Atlantoaxial Fixation Techniques*, Translational Medicine Research, https://doi.org/10.1007/978-981-10-7889-7_16

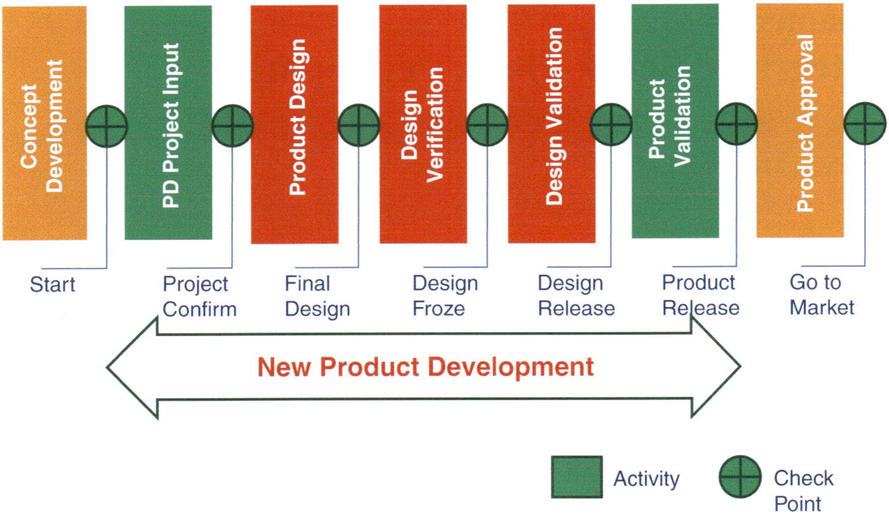

Fig. 16.1 New product development process (Tytus Labs)

16.1.1 *Product Design*

This step transforms clinical needs into prototypes, which requires working with doctors. First, the engineers must transfer clinical requests into a model of the mechanical structure. The model describes the geometrical shape, special location, load distribution, and boundary and restraint conditions of the request. By analyzing the model, engineers then propose an initial design, and use a computer-assisted design (CAD) system to create the basic shape of the product. Most orthopedic products are determined by human anatomy; therefore, the engineers must adjust the shape parameters according to a human body model. Researchers will also perform some basic mechanical analysis and FEM simulations to predict the mechanical properties and structural reliability of the product and then make a prototype using a 3D printing technique. During this step, engineers should have discussions with doctors to predict the function of the products and to determine the surgical steps and tool requirements. After a comparison of several design proposals, the team will choose a final prototype.

16.1.2 *Strength Analysis and Structural Optimization*

After the geometrical shape design is finished, strength analysis must be conducted to ensure the safety of the product. This is done using FEM analysis and structural mechanical experiments. Such experiments include static and dynamic load tests, as well as vibration tests if required. The original design will be modified and optimized according to the analysis and test results. After all parts pass the tests, an assembly will be built to finish whole model optimization and evaluation. However, even if the whole model passes, it is not yet a final design. Further evaluation must be performed to determine whether the product meets the proposed function.

16.1.3 Functional Analysis and Evaluation

After the whole model is finished, the structure's function must be tested to evaluate its effectiveness in the human body. For example, the intended function of a thoracic-lumbar internal fixation system is to restrict the degree of freedom in all directions of spine segments covered by implants. Obviously, the only way to evaluate this is to perform biomechanical tests and calculations. These tests require specific biomechanical facilities, which can capture the motion records of samples, usually using human or animal corpses, while applying loads. During the tests, the samples have two statuses: original status and after-implantation status. The functional analysis will be performed based on the motional differences between these two statuses. Although the tests can demonstrate the proposed function, the results are crude and dispersive because of the functional limitation of the corpse model. It is difficult to evaluate change in internal structures and requires highly skilled operators. Another way to perform biomechanical analysis is computational biomechanical simulations, which apply the same methods stated above on digitized models instead of corpses. Such tests can perform complex and subtle analyses; however, because of uncertainty regarding the parameters of the human body, the results are usually not close to the real samples. Using numerical models is useful to make macroscopic simulations. However, it usually cannot generate precise results. Ultimately, neither test can predict the long-term function of the products because the analysis is static and only represents the short moment the products are implanted. Currently, most biomechanical analysis systems can only acquire motion quantities of samples; therefore, they are mainly used on internal fixation products. Some advanced systems can capture motion modes of samples, which can help to evaluate motive products, such as artificial discs. For these products, live animal test may be performed additionally to evaluate their function.

16.1.4 Surgical Evaluation

In the development of orthopedic products, a suitable set of surgical instruments is an important part of the product. The design of instruments is normally based on specific operational requirements because each step of the operation requires specific instruments. The quality of these instruments determines whether or not the operation can be performed smoothly. To ensure the reliability of the surgical instruments, surgical experiments on cadavers are key. Commonly, this is done by performing the full operation on a cadaver, evaluating the function of each instrument, ensuring that the instruments do not interfere with each other, and brainstorming ideas for further improvement. Based on the results of the cadaver experiment, the design of the instruments is optimized. In addition to cadaver surgery, live animal experiments, model experiments, or computer simulations may also be used to evaluate and enhance surgery.

16.1.5 Design Transfer and Product Validation

After evaluating the mechanical strength and conducting both functional and surgical analyses, a final design is obtained. The next step is to transfer the design to a manufacturer. The manufacturer must construct the manufacture process and tools, choose facilities, control specific process qualities, and establish examination rules, methods, and tests for production. After all these steps are complete, formal production is initiated, and benchmark fatigue tests are performed on random final products. The products will also be sent to related government departments to ensure their safety and effectiveness. The effectiveness evaluation must be passed using clinical experiments. Full documentation covering the development, verification, and validation must be sent and acknowledged by the China Food and Drug Administration (CFDA), after which, the new product can be distributed to the market.

The distribution of the product to the market is the end of pre-development; however, the development of the product continue throughout its life cycle, including product maintenance, design modification, and upgrades.

16.2 Design of the Integrated Screw-Hook System

Initially, Sanyou Medical proposed several drafts of the new atlas-axis posterior fixation system, based on a patent of Changzheng Hospital (Patent No. 200720075767.6). Thereafter, a CAD model was plotted, and assembly of the system with an anatomic spine model was established. The use of surgical instruments was also simulated. Using FEM analysis, the design proposals were optimized, and plastic prototype models were manufactured using 3D printing. The final design drawing was plotted, followed by trial manufacture and mechanical tests. Finally a full-scale evaluation was performed according to all the design proposals.

In the first proposal, a chute was built on the back of the hook to install holders. However, during mechanical tests, the chute significantly decreased the strength of the product. In the following design proposal, a new holding structure was developed so that the chute was no longer necessary (Figs. 16.2 and 16.3). Consequently, the strength increased, and the holding function was still available.

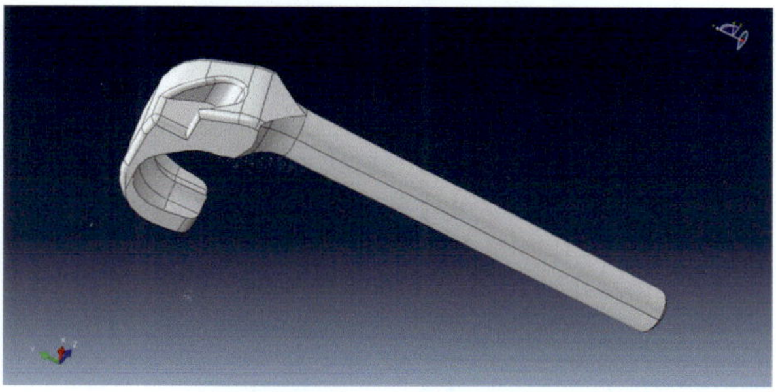

Fig. 16.2 Preliminary design of the hook

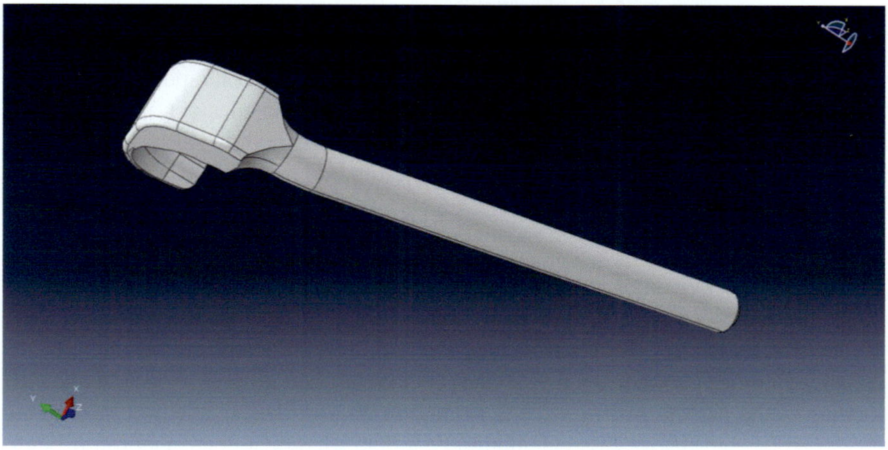

Fig. 16.3 Final design of the hook

16.3 Design Evaluation and Validation

The safety and effectiveness of the novel atlas-axis posterior fixation system were evaluated and confirmed using cadaver experiments, FEM simulations, biomechanical tests, implant strength tests, material biocompatibility tests, and risk assessment evaluation.

16.3.1 Cadaver Surgery

A simulated operation was performed to ensure the intended function of the implants and instruments. The implants were installed smoothly, and the instrument worked well with the implants.

16.3.2 FEM Simulations

An FEM model of the spine was built based on parameters derived from clinical imaging materials. The implant was then installed into the model. Each step was calculated, and stress and displacement analyses were performed. The motion of the original spine model and that of the implanted spine model were compared to predict whether the fixation function worked as intended.

Hypermesh 12.0 performed the preprocess. The setup was as follows:

Interaction
The 13 kinds of key ligaments, anterior atlanto-occipital membrane (AAOM), posterior atlanto-occipital membrane (PAOM), the vertical portion of cruciated ligaments (CLV), apical ligament (AP), alar ligaments (AL), tectorial membrane (TM), transversal ligament (TL), anterior longitudinal ligament (ALL), posterior longitudinal ligament (PLL), ligamentum flavum (LF), facet capsules (FC), interspinous ligament (ISL), and supraspinous ligament (SSL), were modeled as two nodes nonlinear string elements. The contact between joints was modeled as a nonlinear surface to a surface general interaction.

Mesh
Cortical bones were meshed with 1 mm using C3D6 elements, while cancellous bones were meshed using C3D4 elements and an endplate with 0.5 mm C3D6 elements. Intervertebral discs (including the nucleus pulposus) were modeled as enhanced hourglass control C3D8R elements. Hourglass control avoided bulk self-locking in the presence of massive deformation. First-order hexahedron meshes are more precise and invoke less calculation cost than triangle and tetrahedron meshes. Reduced integral elements avoided the hourglass phenomenon, which leads to failure of convergence in massive deformation situations.

Properties The properties of all related materials are shown in Table 16.1.

Loads and Boundary Conditions The boundary condition is complete fix of all six degrees of freedom (DOF) of the bottom endplate of C3. A reference point on the rotation axis of C0 was chosen, and distribution coupling between the point and all nodes on top surface of C0 was established (the load on the point can be transferred to effective pressure on the nodes). A 1.5 Nm torque was applied on the reference point along the X, Y, and Z directions, respectively.

Table 16.1 Material property list

Structure name	Elastic modulus/Mpa	Poisson ratio	Element numbers
Cortical bone	12,000 [4]	0.3	35,208
Cancellous bone	5,000 [5]	0.3	97,588
Endplate	5,000 [5]	0.4	9,088
Titanium	120,000	0.3	

During the simulation, a C0–C3 spine model was first calculated (Fig. 16.4) to obtain the range of motion (ROM) under different actions and compared with reference data, which can be found from Figs. 16.5, 16.6, 16.7, 16.8, 16.9, 16.10, 16.11, 16.12, and 16.13. The results showed that the model was a good representative of real biomechanical structure and was suitable for further implantation evaluation.

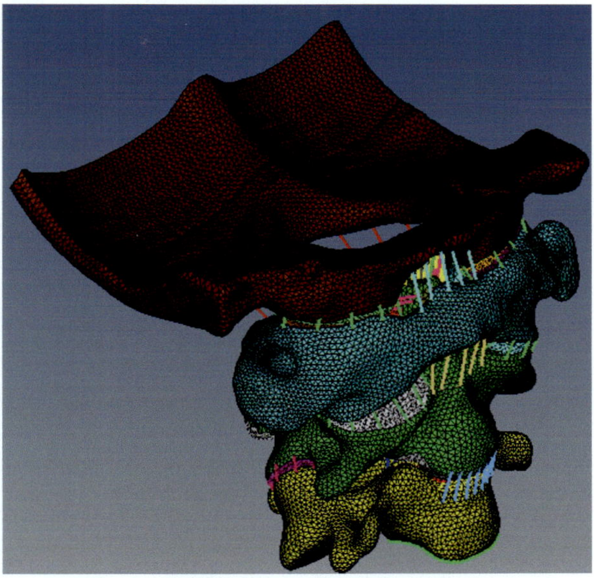

Fig. 16.4 The C0–C3 finite element model

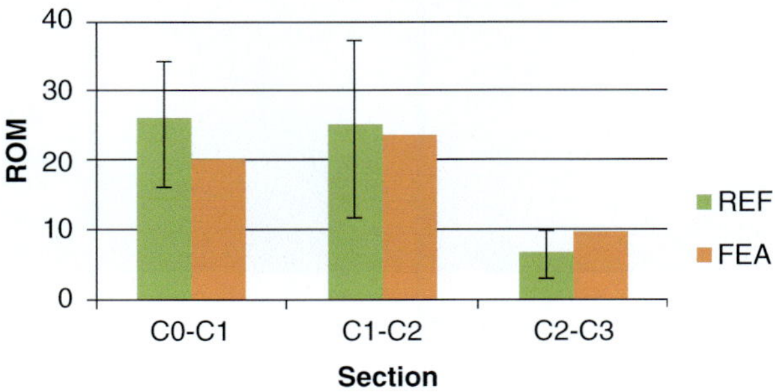

Fig. 16.5 ROM evaluation of flexion and extension

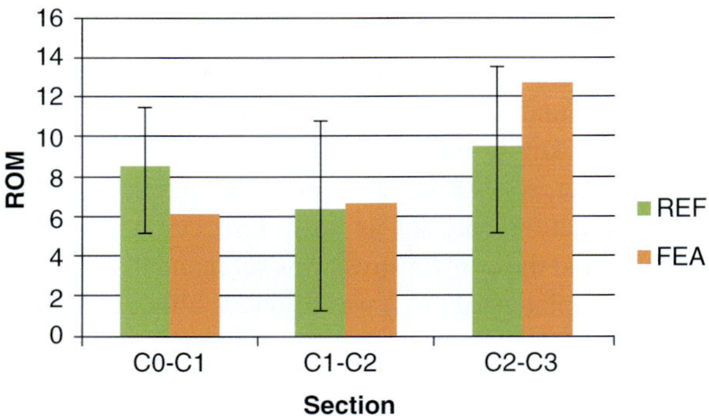

Fig. 16.6 ROM evaluation of left/right bending

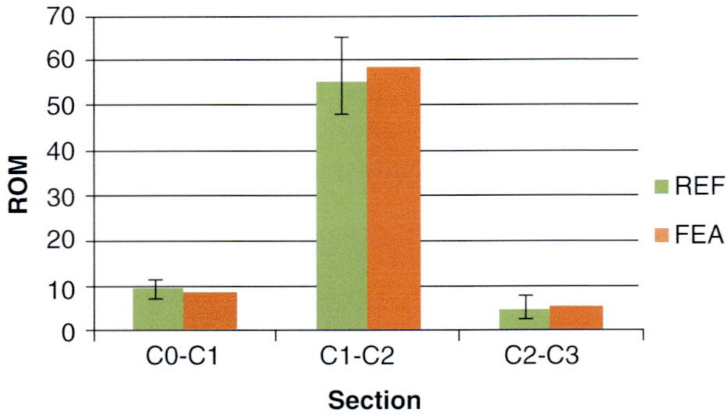

Fig. 16.7 ROM evaluation of left/right torsion

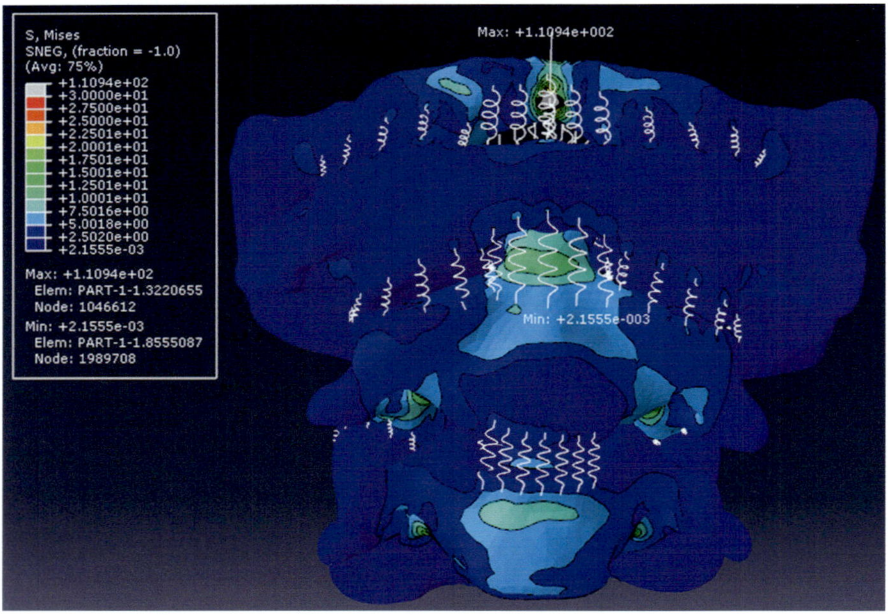

Fig. 16.8 Stress contours of extension

Analysis of biomechanical behavior was performed on different ways of fixation. The fracture model was created by cutting the bottom of the odontoid of the basic model to simulate a type II odontoid fracture. The stability of different fixations was simulated, and ROM and stress contours were plotted.

Several key points of the analysis are: The stress on the endplate was not the main object, so that the element of the endplate was first-order C3D6 and the contact interaction was set as soft. Two contact surfaces can penetrate each other slightly, and the contact stress was set manually. Discontinuity of the stress contours on the endplate (e.g., C2) was allowed, although not for reference.

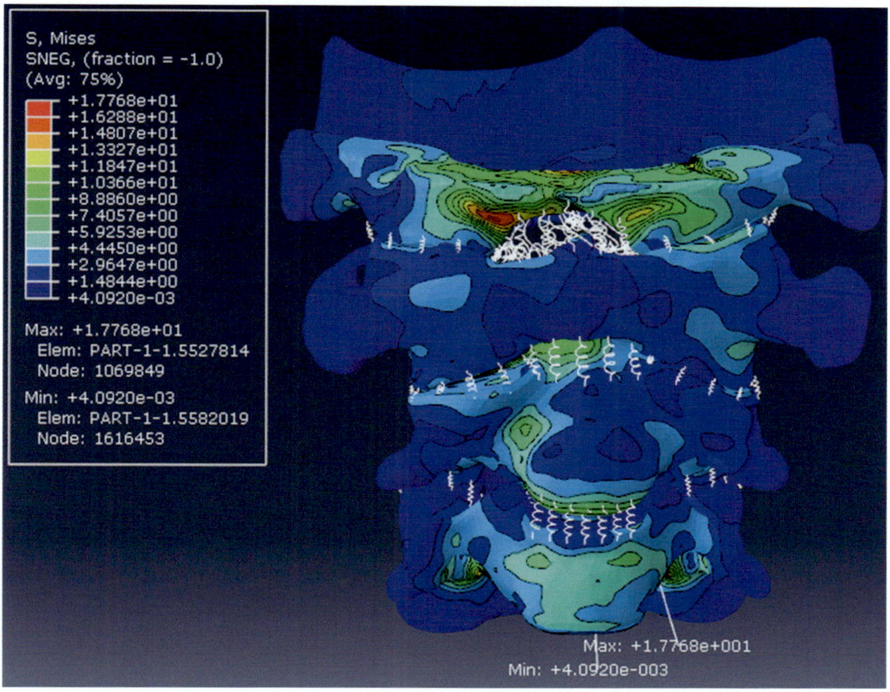

Fig. 16.9 Stress contours of flexion

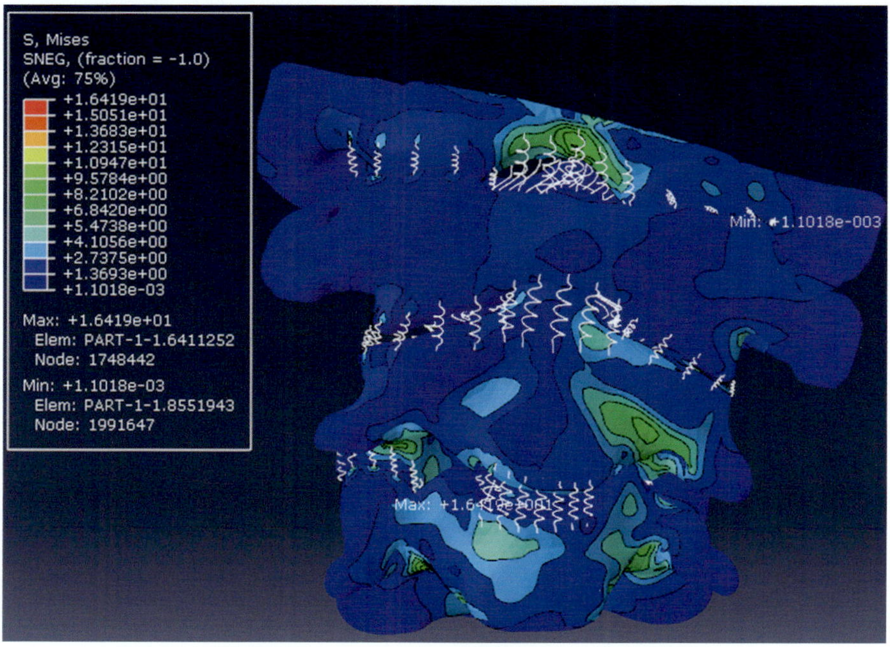

Fig. 16.10 Stress contours of left bending

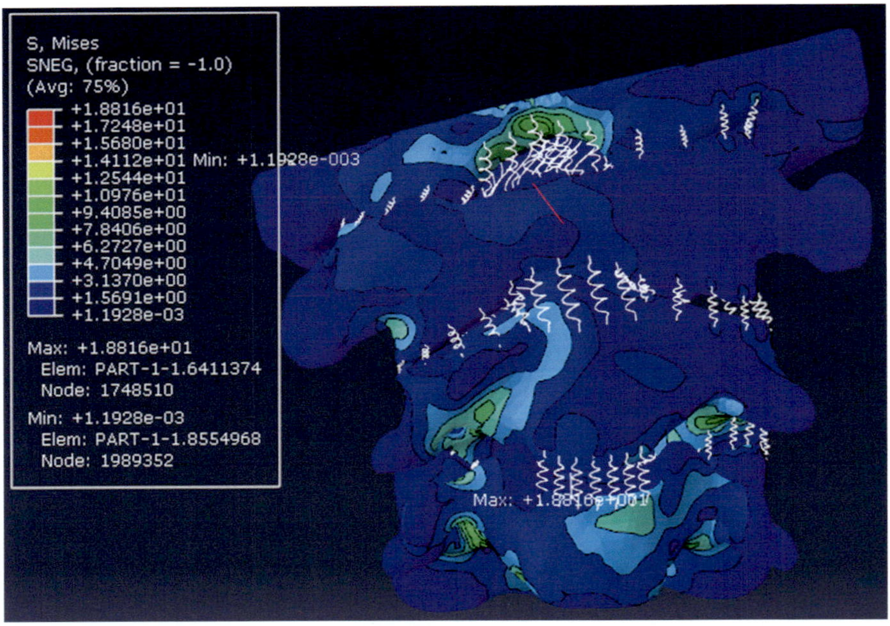

Fig. 16.11 Stress contours of right bending

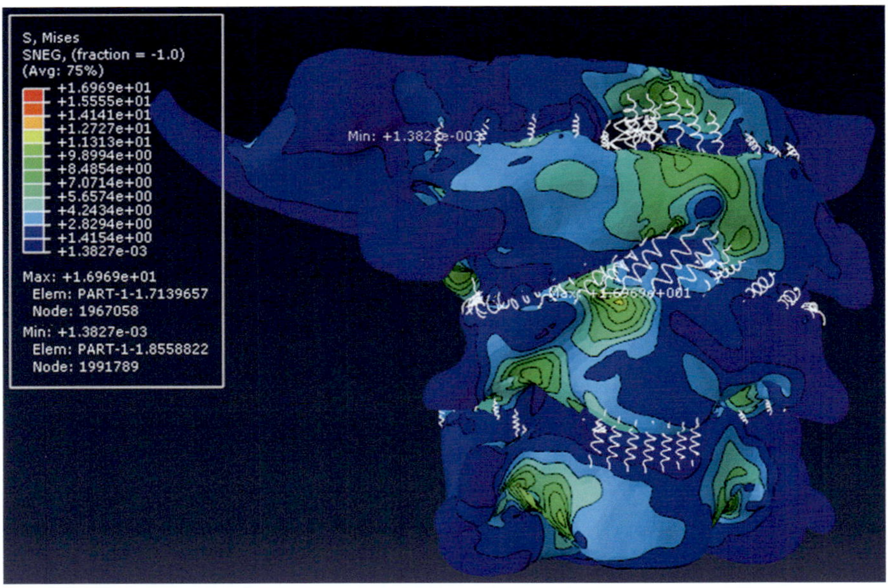

Fig. 16.12 Stress contours of left torsion

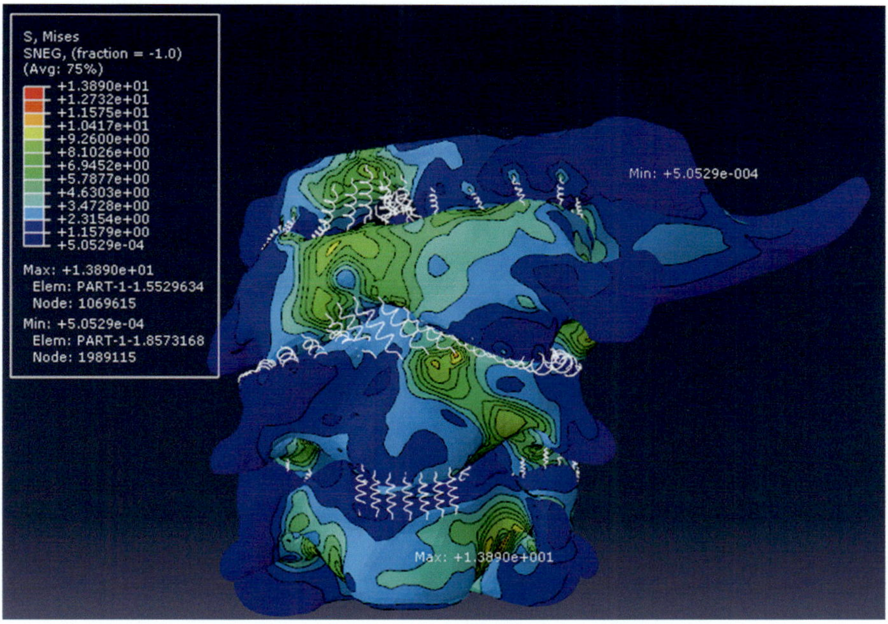

Fig. 16.13 Stress contours of right torsion

When implanting bone chips between C1 and C2, the real interaction was contact and relative slide with each other. Considering the calculation efficiency, a tie interaction was established instead. During calculation, the bone chips would not separate from C1 and C2 and would not show relative displacement.

Although the ligamentum flavum may be partial damaged during bone chip implantation, modeling and simulation showed that the condition would not affect the ROM of C1–C2.

The back part of C0 did not make contact with the head of the pedicle screw because the convergence would be hard to achieve with contact. The real ROM of C0–C1 should be smaller than the calculated value.

Subsequently, different situations of internal fixation systems were modeled (Figs. 16.14, 16.15, 16.16, 16.17, and 16.18), and the ROM was calculated. The results show (Tables 16.2, 16.3, and 16.4) that after the integrated screw-hook was implanted, the total ROM of the atlas-axis structure, especially that of C1–C2, was significantly smaller than that of traditional pedicle screw system. There was an advantage of the system in terms of the stress distribution on the discs (Tables 16.5, 16.6, and 16.7), which made discs bear the least stress. Although the stress distribution of the hook was higher than that of the screw (Tables 16.8, 16.9, and 16.10), it was totally acceptable using the hook structure and suitable material. The simulation proved that the new screw-hook system is superior to previous systems.

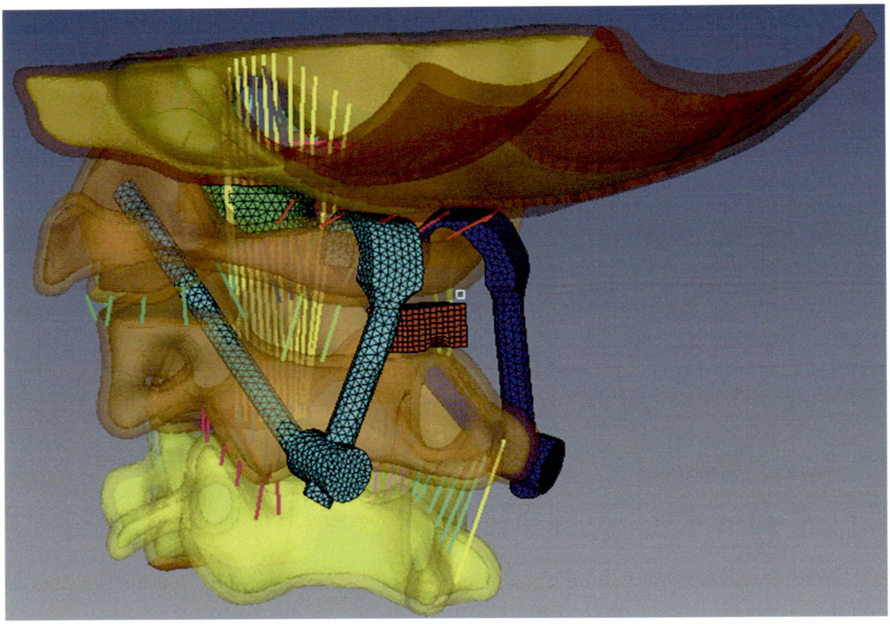

Fig. 16.14 Assembly model of the C1–C2 hook, transarticular screw, and bone chips

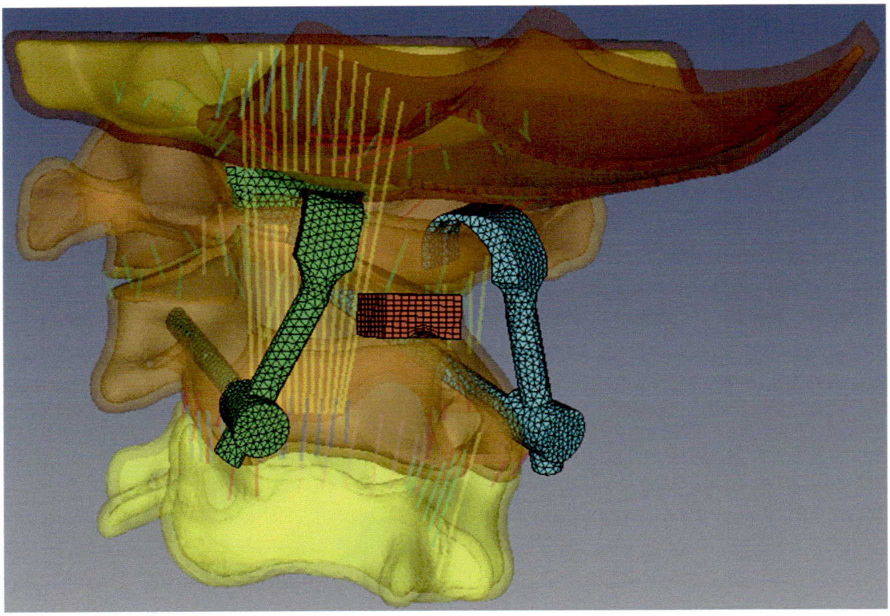

Fig. 16.15 Assembly model of the C1–C2 hook, pedicle screw, and bone chips

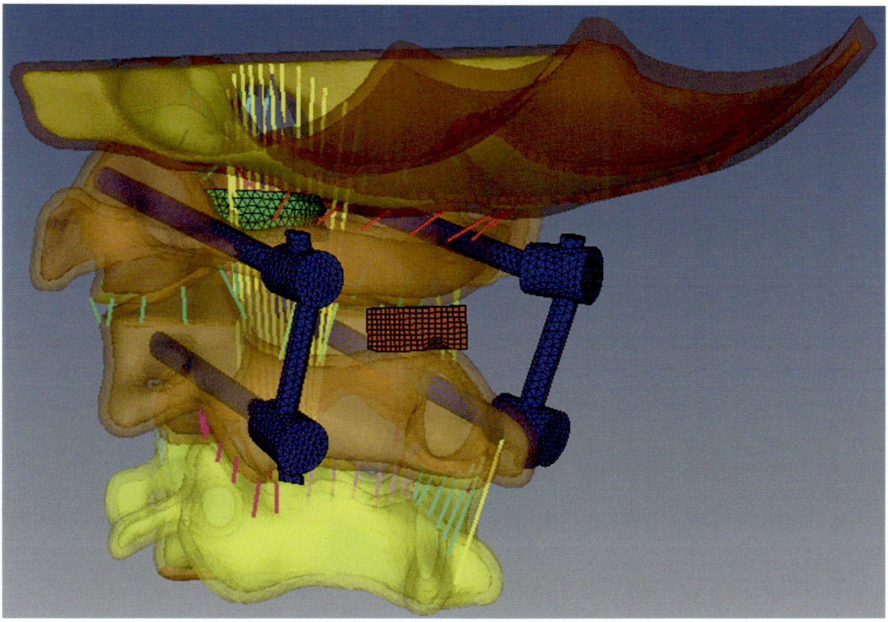

Fig. 16.16 Assembly model of the C1–C2 traditional pedicle screw and bone chips

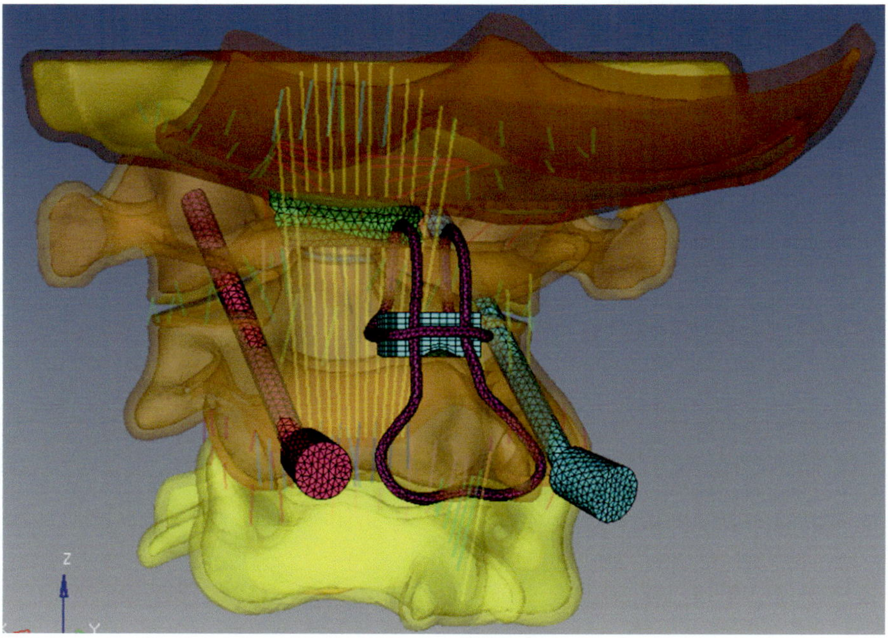

Fig. 16.17 Assembly model of the C1–C2 joint screw, titanium wire, and bone chips

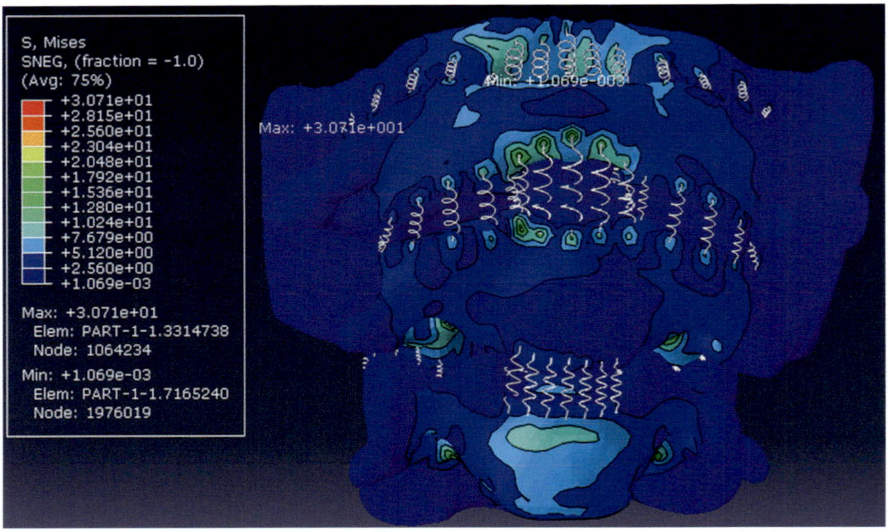

Fig. 16.18 Bone fracture model (fracture of the base of the dentate process retaining the transverse ligament)

Table 16.2 ROM comparisons of flexion and extension

	Flexion + extension		
	C0–C1	C1–C2	C2–C3
Original FEA model	20.27	23.45	9.71
C1–C2 integrated hook-joint screw-bone chips	12.61	0.08	0.33
C1–C2 integrated hook-pedicle screw-bone chips	12.64	0.71	1.03
C1–C2 pedicle screw-bone chips	10.98	1.90	3.25
C1–C2 joint screw-bone chips-titanium wire	12.60	0.11	0.27
Bone fracture model	18.43	36.35	8.48

FEA finite element analysis

Table 16.3 ROM comparison of left/right bending

	Bending (left + right)		
	C0–C1	C1–C2	C2–C3
Original FEA model	6.13	6.68	12.72
C1–C2 integrated hook-joint screw-bone chips	2.01	0.03	0.39
C1–C2 integrated hook-pedicle screw-bone chips	1.97	0.33	1.15
C1–C2 pedicle screw-bone chips	0.80	0.18	0.37
C1–C2 joint screw-bone chips-titanium wire	2.02	0.03	0.28
Bone fracture model	3.7805	7.4969	12.7236

FEA finite element analysis

Table 16.4 ROM comparison of left/right torsion

	Torsion (left + right)		
	C0–C1	C1–C2	C2–C3
Original FEA model	9.60	58.34	5.59
C1–C2 integrated hook-joint screw-bone chips	3.18	0.02	0.42
C1–C2 integrated hook-pedicle screw-bone chips	3.21	0.16	0.84
C1–C2 pedicle screw-bone chips	4.80	6.58	2.85
C1–C2 joint screw-bone chips-titanium wire	3.17	0.04	0.37
Bone fracture model	9.59	59.26	5.63

FEA finite element analysis

16.3.3 Biomechanical Experiments

Table 16.5 Maximum stress of intervertebral discs (flexion and extension)

	Flexion	Extension
	C2–C3	C2–C3
Original FEA model	3.73	5.87
C1–C2 integrated hook-joint screw-bone chips	0.86	0.49
C1–C2 integrated hook-pedicle screw-bone chips	1.54	0.88
C1–C2 pedicle screw-bone chips	5.53	3.61
C1–C2 joint screw-bone chips-titanium wire	0.82	0.47
Bone fracture model	5.87	3.68

FEA finite element analysis

Six fresh C1–C3 specimens were selected, and the bottom of C3 was fixed onto the

Table 16.6 Maximum stress of intervertebral discs (left/right bending)

	Left lateral bending	Right lateral bending
	C2–C3	C2–C3
Original FEA model	3.11	3.47
C1–C2 integrated hook-joint screw-bone chips	0.52	0.55
C1–C2 integrated hook-pedicle screw-bone chips	0.73	0.77
C1–C2 pedicle screw-bone chips	3.07	3.42
C1–C2 joint screw-bone chips-titanium wire	0.49	0.56
Bone fracture model	3.14	3.48

FEA finite element analysis

Table 16.7 Maximum stress of intervertebral discs (left/right torsion)

	Left torsion C2–C3	Right torsion C2–C3
Original FEA model	2.68	3.55
C1–C2 integrated hook-joint screw-bone chips	0.78	0.86
C1–C2 integrated hook-pedicle screw-bone chips	1.25	1.35
C1–C2 pedicle screw-bone chips	2.68	3.55
C1–C2 joint screw-bone chips-titanium wire	0.75	0.81
Bone fracture model	2.68	3.56

FEA finite element analysis

biomechanical test machine. A static load of 50 N was applied to the top surface of C1, and C1 was moved as follows: extend and flex, bend left and right, and the

Table 16.8 Maximum stress of the fixation system (flexion and extension)

	Flexion	Extension
C1–C2 integrated hook-joint screw-bone chips	283.9	328.6
C1–C2 integrated hook-pedicle screw-bone chips	167.7	171.7
C1–C2 pedicle screw-bone chips	97.76	122.9
C1–C2 joint screw-bone chips-titanium wire	58.35	46.37

Table 16.9 Maximum stress of the fixation system (left/right bending)

	Left lateral bending	Right lateral bending
C1–C2 integrated hook-joint screw-bone chips	388.4	380.9
C1–C2 integrated hook-pedicle screw-bone chips	153.6	149.3
C1–C2 pedicle screw-bone chips	117.0	103.6
C1–C2 joint screw-bone chips-titanium wire	21.04	28.28

Table 16.10 Maximum stress of the fixation system (left/right torsion)

	Left torsion	Right torsion
C1–C2 integrated hook-joint screw-bone chips	445.0	424.3
C1–C2 integrated hook-pedicle screw-bone chips	129.3	180.7
C1–C2 pedicle screw-bone chips	119.7	120.6
C1–C2 joint screw-bone chips-titanium wire	22.32	22.34

application of axial torsion. The amplitude was set at 7 Nm, with increasing increments of 1 Nm. All displacements occurring in each direction (three direction displacements and three axial rotations) were recorded, and 18 load-displacement curves were plotted. The implants were added and the experiments were repeated. Finally, the motion behaviors of the two specimens were compared to determine whether the system could provide proper stability.

16.3.4 Mechanical Experiments on the Implants

The implants were fixed on the static and dynamic test machines, and static and dynamic loads were applied on the implants to simulate worst-case scenarios. The static load was applied until the implant failed. The dynamic load was applied at a frequency of 5 Hz until the implant failed or the loading cycle reached 5 million times. In the dynamic test, if an implant failed, the amplitude of load was decreased, and the test was repeated until the implants passed 5 million cycles of loading, which is termed the fatigue strength. These tests ensured the reliability of the product.

16.3.5 Biocompatibility Test of Materials

A standard biocompatibility test was introduced during the design to make sure the materials used for the implants do not harm the human body.

16.3.6 Risk Assessment Evaluation of Design

Risk assessment was performed such that the design met the requirements of global, domestic, and industrial standards.

16.4 Industrial Production Process and Product Quality Control

After the product was designed and verified, we determined the production and processing technology, which included processing methods, production methods, equipment choice, and the design and manufacture of accessories. By setting up a process control system and related documentation, we determined the product specification and standards and the design and manufacturing tools. A series of standard orthopedic experiments were conducted on the finished product after it passed the capability test. Security and reliability were ensured by standard static and fatigue tests on random samples of the first batch of finished products.

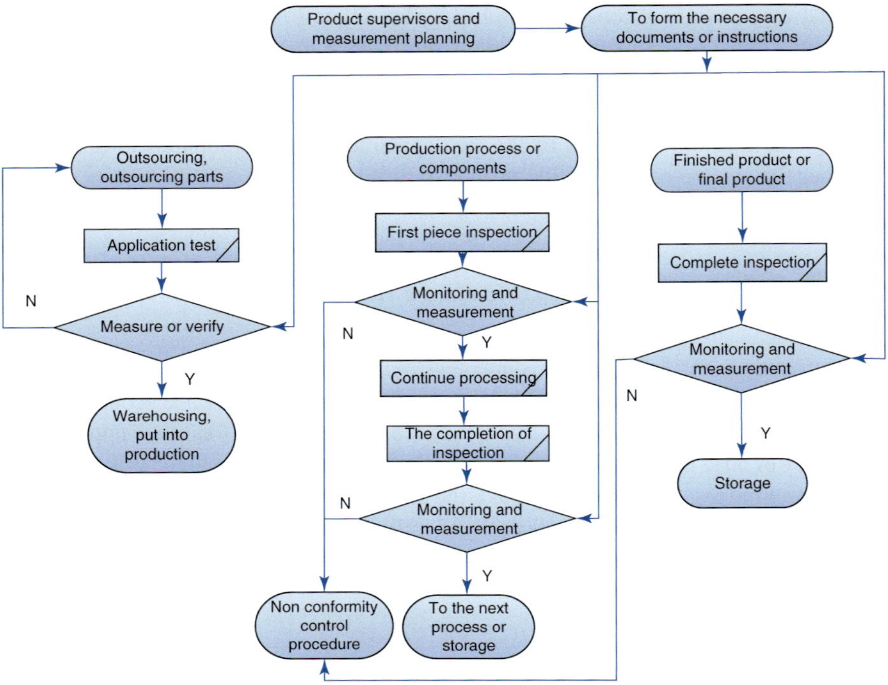

Fig. 16.19 Production flow chart of Sanyou Medical

After the overall risk evaluation was performed and the product technical documentation was completed, we obtained a third-party medical device testing report, which was authenticated by the CFDA. This marked the end of the product research and development process by both hospital and the company. The project then proceeded to mass production and initial clinical use phase (Fig. 16.19).

The quality control department of the company performed spot checks in accordance with the relevant standards and regulations [6].

References

1. Title 21-Food and drugs, Chapter I-Food and drug administration, Department of Health and Human Services, Subchapter H-medical devices, Subpart C-design controls, § 820.30–Design controls.
2. ISO 13485:2016, Medical devices-Quality management systems-Requirements for regulatory purposes.
3. Council directive 93/42/EEC of 14 June 1993 concerning medical devices.
4. Shirazi-Adl A, Ahmed AM, Shrivastava SC. Mechanical response of a lumbar motion segment in axial torque alone and combined with compression. Spine. 1986;11(9):914–27.
5. Schmidt H, Heuer F, Drumm J, Klezl Z, Claes L, Wilke HJ. Application of a calibration method provides more realistic results for a finite element model of a lumbar spinal segment. Clin Biomech (Bristol, Avon). 2007;22(4):377–84.
6. Regulation of Quality Control Department in Sanyou Medical, Quality Control Department, Shanghai Sanyou Co., Ltd. 2011.

Chapter 17
Putting the Integrated Screw-Hook System on the Market

Michael Mingyan Liu

Abstract The integrated screw-hook system will be used mainly to treat upper cervical lesions, more precisely, atlantoaxial fixation to stabilize the atlas and axis. Currently, the main products used to treat upper cervical spine patients are screw-rod fixation and screw-hook fixation systems, such as the Vertex and Cervrina systems. The integrated screw-hook system combines the advantages of the screw-rod fixation and screw-hook fixation systems. The atlantoaxial fixation market is a small but indispensable market segment, which fills the blank and has a unique competitive status in this market segment. The product life cycle can be divided into four stages: introduction, growth, maturity, and recession. We received good feedback during early clinical use. Short-term follow-up results showed that the method has advantages of strong internal fixation, a high rate of bone graft, and an obvious curative effect.

17.1 Market Analysis and Expected Product Life Cycle

The integrated screw-hook system will be used mainly to treat upper cervical lesions, more precisely, atlantoaxial fixation to stabilize the atlas and axis. Many factors contribute to the development of upper cervical lesions, including trauma, tumors, infections, congenital malformations, degenerative diseases, and rheumatoid arthritis. The resulting instability causes pillow neck pain and severe injuries to the cervical spinal cord, which can be fatal. Atlantoaxial instability can be divided into acute and chronic instability; arthrodesis consists of anterior fusion and posterior fusion. It mainly applies to:

1. Transverse ligament rupture
2. Type II fracture of the dentate process, except screw fixation of the dens
3. Odontoid atlantoaxial instability caused by odontoid dysplasia or isolated bone

M. M. Liu
Shanghai Sanyou Medical Co. Ltd, Shanghai, China
e-mail: mingyan.liu@sanyou-medical.com

B. Ni et al. (eds.), *Atlantoaxial Fixation Techniques*, Translational Medicine Research, https://doi.org/10.1007/978-981-10-7889-7_17

4. Destruction of the vertebral body caused by tuberculosis or a tumor of the upper cervical spine
5. Instability of the atlas and axis or severe pain in the occipital and neck caused by rheumatoid arthritis
6. Transverse ligament and joint capsule ligament relaxation or atlantoaxial instability caused by local infection

Atlantoaxial surgery is very difficult and high risk because of the complicated anatomical structure and abundance of the nerve and vascular tissue surrounding the area. Currently, this kind of surgery is almost exclusively carried out in 3A hospitals, thus making it a specialized and indispensable market.

In an attempt to reduce the risk and complications of upper cervical spine surgery and to allow more hospitals to perform such operations, many surgeons and orthopedic companies have devoted much time and resources to the study of atlantoaxial fusion and internal fixation in the last 10 years, resulting in some progress.

Atlantoaxial fusion surgery includes posterior fusion and anterior fusion. Anterior fusion consists of Magerl screw fixation and fusion with trans-oral anterior screw fixation. However, this technique is rarely used in clinical applications because of the difficulty of atlantoaxial exposure and the high risks of injuring the superior laryngeal nerve and inferior lingual nerve.

Posterior atlantoaxial fusion is the most common method because of its clear atlantoaxial exposure and ease of operation. The internal fixation products for posterior atlantoaxial fusion consist of cables, clips (hooks), atlantoaxial transarticular screws, stick systems, and hook systems.

The most representative cable bundle-fixed fusions are the Gallie and Brooks techniques. The Brooks technique uses two double steel wires through the posterior arch of the atlas and the lamina of the axis, taking in two iliac cortical zones, pruning after planting on both sides of the midline, and tying with wire. Its fixed points are on the posterior arch of the atlas and the lamina; therefore, the Brooks technique has higher biomechanical stability than the Gallie technique. Aside from strengthening anti-flexion and back extension, it can also constrain the limits of atlantoaxial rotation and lateral flexion partially. However, it cannot control the translational motion between the atlantoaxial; the failure rate remains as high as 30% and is much worse in the treatment of fractures of the dens and transverse rupture of the transverse ligament. Its lack of mechanical stability means that cable fixing needs halo vest fastening for 12 weeks to limit the atlantoaxial rotational and translational motion to ensure bone fusion. In addition, the wire cuts through the lamina of the axis, carrying a high risk of injuring the cervical spinal cord, and is rarely used in the treatment of atlantoaxial dislocation.

As an improvement to the cable bundling fixed fusion, atlantoaxial interspinous fixation devices, such as the Apofix system, have been applied widely in upper cervical fixation. However, interspinous fixation is still a type of two-point fixation, which cannot avoid the poor control of rotary stress and the uncontrollability of translation. It still needs to be maintained with strong external fixation and requires the completion of the posterior arch of the atlas. From a product cycle aspect, interspinous fixation has gone through the publishing period, introduction period, and growing period but has gone into the decline phase without a maturation period. Currently, the Apofix system is delisted.

Atlantoaxial transarticular screw fixation was developed at the same time as the Apofix system. Magerl and Seeman used bilateral transarticular screw fixation for atlantoaxial instability in 1987, which visibly reduced the occurrence of pseudarthrosis and bone nonunion. It was reported that the bone fusion rate was 95–100%. In the Magerl technology, a screw goes through the atlantoaxial joint to the lateral mass of the atlas, while connecting atlantoaxial joint center on both sides, close to the diameter of atlas. It comprises central fixation, whose anti-rotation, anti-lateriflexion, and anti-shearing forces are better, but remains poor in terms of the anti-bending force. The main advantages of Magerl technology are:

1. No need for a halo vest, neck support is enough.
2. It does not depend on the integrity of the posterior arch and can help to reduce pressure on the posterior arch of the atlas and the lamina of the axis.
3. No wire goes under posterior arch of the atlas and the lamina of the axis, which reduces damage to the spinal cord and nerves.

Magerl technology is suitable for patients with inflammatory lesions or spinal cord diseases caused by pannus formation. Although still on the market, Magerl technology has a small market share because of its limited market application resulting from excessive complications and risks, as well as high operating requirements.

Currently, the main products used to treat upper cervical spine patients are screw-rod fixation and screw-hook fixation systems, such as the Vertex and Cervrina systems. Screw-rod fixation connects the ipsilateral lateral mass screw of the atlas and the axis pedicle screw symmetrically with the tail-side connection.

Screw-hook fixation is performed by first inserting a screw through the joint space, selecting appropriate C1 lamina hook using a lamina test model, connecting the same side Magerl screw and a C1 lamina hook nail tail with a connecting rod, and repeating the procedure on the other side. Using a shaped autogenous iliac bone block embedded in the C1 back arch and the C2 spike process, the bone graft is fixed firmly by the longitudinal pressure of the connecting rod. Although bilateral atlantoaxial transarticular screws and C1 laminar hook fixation are not specifically designed for upper cervical spine surgery due to its on anatomy and disregard for the specific requirements of upper cervical spine surgery, this kind of internal fixation is a type of tri-point fixation, which has high biomechanical stability and good control of atlantoaxial flexion, lateral flexion, and rotation. It is a practical and effective atlantoaxial fusion internal fixation system that helps patients move freely earlier and also has a higher fusion success rate. These are the main competitive products for the integrated screw-hook system.

The integrated screw-hook system combines the advantages of the screw-rod fixation and screw-hook fixation systems. There is no need to pass through posterior fixation in atlantoaxial vertebral lamina, which is a relatively easy procedure. Atlas laminar hooks and atlantoaxial transarticular screws are connected, which combine the tri-point fixation and compressive bone graft into one system. It overcomes the weakness of Magerl screw resilience and fully reflects the concept of three-dimensional fixation of atlantoaxial biomechanics. The integrated screw-hook system is also specifically designed for upper cervical spine surgery. Remarkably, the large angle screw designed for C2's special anatomy can be implanted directly and perfectly fits C2's anatomy, which greatly reduces the fixation system structure of the rod notch. The integrated screw-hook system is also designed carefully to fit the C1 and prevents the hook C1 "wiper" effect. These features all contribute to the stability of internal fixation and provide unique competitive advantage to the product on the market.

As far as the whole spinal market is concerned, thoracolumbar spine surgery accounts for 52%, and cervical vertebra surgery accounts for about 48%. From a sales perspective, thoracolumbar spine products (including thoracic and lumbar interbody fusion) have about 70% of the market, while cervical vertebra and cervical fusion only account for about 25%, and posterior cervical fixation systems account for a mere 5% of the entire market. Disregarding the cervical intervertebral fusion device market share and subdividing cervical posterior fixation systems into two categories, cervical atlantoaxial fixation accounts for only 1%. Thus, the atlantoaxial fixation market is a small but indispensable market segment. The integrated screw-hook system fills the blank and has a unique competitive status in this market segment.

17.2 Product Life Cycle of the Integrated Screw-Hook System

The product life cycle can be divided into four stages: introduction, growth, maturity, and recession. The integrated screw-hook system is obviously superior to the common cervical posterior screw-hook system, which should show rapid sales growth in introduction period. Those surgeons who have been looking for an internal fixation device dedicated to the upper cervical spine will be keen on the integrated screw-hook system and will be keen to put it into clinical application. The rapid spread of the product and sales growth may make us think of a "social trend" life cycle, that is, quick recession after outbreak. However, the actual situation should be different because the currently most common cervical screw-hook system is significantly less effective than the integrated screw-hook system, suggesting that the integrated system will become somewhat irreplaceable. Thus, we infer that the sales curve will extend within a small range without slumping in the growth and maturity periods. This represents the so-called "styled" product life cycle. This kind of life cycle is driven not only by its irreplaceable character but also by the mass quantity of potential customers, who have been concerned about the difficulty and risk of the surgery in the absence of a good upper cervical spine internal fixation system. These customers will have the confidence to use integrated screw-hook system to cure atlantoaxial dislocation after product training. In other words, if the product becomes a kind of culture and trend, through a variety of market incentives and product training, our system would continue selling for a long period before going into the recession period.

17.3 Early Clinical Use and Feedback for the Integrated Screw-Hook System

We received good feedback during early clinical use. Short-term follow-up results showed that the method has advantages of strong internal fixation, a high rate of bone graft, and an obvious curative effect. All cases showed bone fusion, and no strong external fixation was needed. Designing the system specifically according to the upper cervical atlantoaxial anatomy of Chinese patients allowed the system to overcome the problems associated with previous hook systems, such as Vertex. In addition, the fact that the instrument system was designed specifically for upper cervical spine surgery makes the installation process relatively simple and reduces the operation time and the amount of bleeding.

All patients had smooth operations, without spinal cord injuries, or damage to nerve roots or the vertebral artery. The amount of bleeding was low, and the operation time was relatively short. Postoperatively, the patients' spinal cord function improved, and their limb numbness and inability symptoms were relieved. All patients obtained bone fusion without loosening of the internal fixation screw breaking or re-dislocation. There was also no cerebral ischemia or other operation-related symptoms.

Otherwise, from the feedback during early clinical use, although the integrated screw-hook system brought better atlantoaxial reduction and easier surgery, an appropriate method of bone grafting and immediate postoperative stability are the key to the success of atlantoaxial fusion. With improvements in surgical techniques and internal fixation devices, the atlantoaxial fusion success rate will improve, and complications will decrease significantly. Meanwhile, early rehabilitation training is also very important, as it would reduce the need for long-term external fixation. The complexity of the axial root structure and the high risk of surgery require surgeons to develop a careful plan according to the specific circumstances of the patient's and select a safe and effective way of integration.

In summary, the new integrated screw-hook system combines the advantages of the joint screw technology and the lamina hook technique. It is a practical and effective atlantoaxial fusion internal fixation system that achieves anterior and posterior internal fixation and pressure bone graft simultaneously, which fully reflects the concept of three-dimensional fixation of atlantoaxial biomechanics.

MIX
Papier aus verantwortungsvollen Quellen
Paper from responsible sources
FSC® C105338

If you have any concerns about our products,
you can contact us on
ProductSafety@springernature.com

In case Publisher is established outside the EU,
the EU authorized representative is:
Springer Nature Customer Service Center GmbH
Europaplatz 3, 69115 Heidelberg, Germany

Printed by Libri Plureos GmbH
in Hamburg, Germany